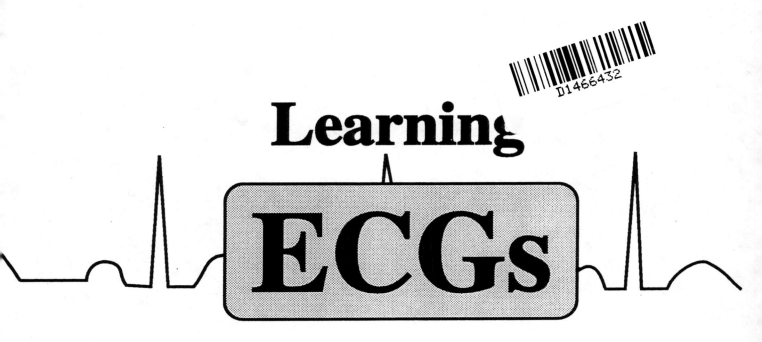

Learning ECGs

INSTRUCTOR'S MANUAL

WRITTEN BY

CINDY TAIT
RN, BS, CEN, CCRN

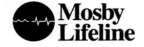

Mosby
Lifeline

An Affiliate of Elsevier Science

St. Louis   London   Philadelphia   Sydney   Toronto

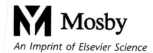

Mosby

An Imprint of Elsevier Science

Editor: Claire Merrick
Developmental Editor: Ross Goldberg
Project Manager: Peggy Fagen
Manufacturing Supervisor: Patricia Stinecipher

Mosby, Inc.
11830 Westline Industrial Drive
St. Louis, Missouri 63146

International Standard Book Number 0-8016-8095-6

02 03 04 05 06 /PC 9 8 7 6 5 4 3 2

TABLE OF CONTENTS

HOW TO USE THIS MANUAL

This instructor's manual closely correlates with the video series and student workbook. It has been designed to assist you with planning and presenting the course content, as well as evaluating your students' comprehension of the subject. The study of ECG interpretation is a large entity. You may want to supplement the information in this manual based on your experience as a teacher. Feel free to be creative and adapt the material according to your teaching style and the classroom situation.

Each video tape has the capacity to "stand alone" and provides adequate information to comprehensively cover the given topic. However, it is recommended that the information be presented in order, as many of the basic principles presented in the first tapes are expounded upon later in the series. Also, insure adequate learning of each lesson before moving on. Your students will have a greater motivation to pursue the next lesson if they receive positive feedback from the instructor and have successfully completed the lesson in the student workbook.

You may want to present the video at the beginning of the lesson, or after an introductory lecture covering the key points that will be presented. Watch the video with your students and be prepared to answer questions and elaborate on the topic. You may want to stop the tape at designated intervals to discuss and review the information. Your students may appreciate the opportunity to borrow the videos for additional review. Students will benefit from the repetition of information and learner anxiety may be reduced by viewing the tape at their own pace outside of the classroom setting.

Each chapter in this manual provides you with a lesson plan for the video tape of the same title. Included in each chapter are:

Goals which will assist you in familiarizing yourself with the content of each lesson prior to classroom presentation.

Learning objectives to help place the topic in perspective and to acquaint the student with the information that will be presented. Learner expectations and goals are clarified prior to each lesson.

Outlines which provide a synopsis of the information presented in each video. Content is then divided into topics and smaller subdivisions. Following the outline will allow you to present the information in the same sequence as the video tape.

Vocabulary lists identify terms as they are introduced to the student. The science of cardiology is replete with a multitude of terms and abbreviations that may be new to your students. You may want to test your students' comprehension by asking them to define or use these words in their proper context. Appendix A provides a glossary of the terms listed in each lesson.

Review questions place key points from each video in question form. Student learning can be monitored by asking review questions prior to advancing to the next lesson.

Case studies are provided to allow practice identifying rhythms. Each case study includes a scenario and related rhythm strip to stimulate group discussion regarding assessment and management of patients with dysrhythmias.

The five appendices include:

A - Glossary of terms - defines commonly used terms related to ECG interpretation and care of cardiac patients. This appendix can be distributed as a handout or used for review and testing.

B - Common cardiac medications - lists commonly prescribed medications for the treatment of the dysrhythmias and diseases covered in the series.

C - Cardiac assessment - defines the basic parameters for assessing cardiac patients. It is offered as a guide for assessing patient tolerance of acute and chronic dysrhythmias.

D - Transparency masters - are provided to use as a classroom adjunct, or as handouts to supplement the videos and student workbook.

E - Annotated bibliography - recommends supplemental readings related to ECG interpretation and patient management. This guide will be useful for students or instructors seeking information beyond the basic curricula provided in this series. A brief description of each text is provided and recommendations made as to the content level.

Should you have any questions or concerns regarding the video tapes or materials provided in this series, please contact us at American Safety Video Publishers (1-800-722-2572) so that we may respond to your inquiries.

TEACHING STRATEGIES

Before delving into the individual lessons, let's review some basic learning theories and teaching strategies. Adult learners typically enter educational experiences with a motivation to learn. Their intent is to gain knowledge and skills that are pertinent to their lives and careers. Your students will bring to class a variety of interests, attitudes, values, and previous learning experiences. It is the challenge of the instructor to meet the student at this reference point and to create an environment optimal to the learning process.

Learning can be defined as a process of change through which people acquire new knowledge, skills or attitudes as a result of some type of study or experience. Learning is the responsibility of the student and requires a choice to apply one's energies toward assimilating information and acquiring skills. Learners must come to class with a readiness to learn, as success in learning is directly proportional to student motivation.

There are three domains of learning: cognitive, psychomotor and affective. Cognitive learning involves giving information to students via lecture, video tapes, written materials, etc. Psychomotor learning requires the student to have a base of knowledge and the neuromuscular ability to perform a given skill. Affective learning requires student motivation, the direct result being a change in attitude, enthusiasm, belief, confidence and/or sense of commitment to learning and to the subject matter.

An effective instructor is a leader, as learning is more often "caught than taught". It is the responsibility of the instructor to be knowledgeable in the topic and to impart that knowledge in an organized, well planned and concise manner. Learning is more easily accomplished when the instructor is confident with the material and presents the information with enthusiasm in a friendly and nonthreatening environment.

Learning Principles

Motivation - Show enthusiasm for the subject matter. Make learning a fun and exciting experience. Offer students recognition and respect. This will result in a reciprocal respect for the instructor and subject matter.

Repetition - Frequent review and practice will reinforce learning. Remember that it is not "practice that makes perfect," but rather, "perfect practice that makes perfect" - this requires structured practice and continuous feedback.

Use of senses - Learning is best accomplished when the information is seen, heard and done. In addition to the videos and workbook, encourage student participation with activities such as: study groups, case studies, role playing and skills demonstrations.

Association - Word association using rhymes or mnemonics may help with memorization of facts or sequences of information.

Structure - Sequential presentation of information from simple to complex enhances learning. This requires the instructor to plan and organize the information in a progressive manner.

Feedback - Knowledge of success is a motivation for continued learning and encourages the learner to move forward to more complex information and higher levels of competency. Feedback needs to be timely, and can quickly correct misconceptions and misinformation. Learner anxiety is reduced and learning reinforced when positive feedback is offered.

Evaluation - Student progress can be evaluated by many methods. A few examples are observation, interview, and written or oral examinations. A positive evaluation will motivate the student to continue learning.

Emotions -Learning can be threatening. Contributing factors can be perceived pressure from peers or employers, fear of failure, perfectionism or previous negative learning experiences. A good instructor can overcome these obstacles by adopting a non-prejudicial, non-judgmental attitude toward students. Instructors can establish a non-threatening atmosphere by being approachable and maintaining communication that is friendly, warm and encouraging.

Applicability - Students desire infomation that will assist them in their practices. Introduce topics with a "need to know" explanation, and whenever possible, apply the information as it relates to patient care.

Problem Solving - Ultimate learning is accomplished when the student has assimilated the information to a level that allows him or her to solve real-life problems. Providing the students with real-life patient problems will allow you to evaluate their level of learning.

Best regards as you share this information with your students.

ANATOMY AND PHYSIOLOGY OF THE HEART

GOALS

After completing this lesson the student will be able to demonstrate knowledge of:

◊ the basic anatomical stuctures of the heart.

◊ the location of the heart and its relationship to the other structures within the thoracic cavity.

◊ the route of blood flow through the heart, lungs and circulatory system.

◊ normal and abnormal heart sounds.

◊ the location and function of the coronary arteries.

◊ the action potential of myocardial cells.

◊ the electrical conduction system within the myocardium.

◊ the normal P,Q,R,S,T waveforms as displayed on the ECG tracing.

◊ the influence of the autonomic nervous system on the strength, rate and force of the heart.

◊ the relationship between electrical conduction and mechanical contraction of the heart.

◊ the properties of automaticity and conductivity.

◊ the two primary functions of blood.

◊ the principles of strength and stretch of the myocardium as they relate to preload.

OBJECTIVES

◊ Explain the importance of ECG interpretation as a component of cardiac care.

◊ Label the basic anatomical structures of the heart.

◊ Discuss the relationship between electrical conduction and mechanical contraction within the myocardium.

◊ Trace the route of blood as it passes through each valve and chamber of the heart.

◊ State the three layers of the myocardium and the function of each.

◊ Describe the phases of systole and diastole as they apply to the filling and pumping of the heart.

◊ State the names and locations of the four cardiac valves.

◊ Correlate normal and abnormal heart sounds with the ECG tracing.

◊ Discuss the structure and function of arteries and veins.

◊ Describe the movement of electrolytes as they move across the myocardial cell membrane during depolarization.

◊ Identify each portion of the electrical conduction system from the SA node to the Purkinje fibers.

◊ Correlate the P,Q,R,S,T waveforms with the location of electrical stimulation within the cardiac conduction system.

◊ State two important functions of blood.

◊ Identify the portions of the myocardium and electrical conduction system supplied by each of the coronary arteries.

OUTLINE

I. Introduction

A. Cardiac Anatomy and Physiology

B. Coronary Circulation

C. Electrical Conduction System

D. Autonomic Nervous System

II. Anatomy of the Heart

A. Size

B. Location
   1. Surrounding structures

C. Pericardium
   1. Three layers
   2. Protective fluid

D. Function

E. Structures
   1. Atria
   2. Ventricles
   3. AV valves
      a. tricuspid
      b. mitral
   4. Semilunar valves
      a. aortic
      b. pulmonic

F. Heart Sounds
   1. Normal
   2. Abnormal

III. Circulation

A. Pulmonary
   1. Oxygen/carbon dioxide exchange

B. Systemic
   1. Arteries and veins
      a. tunica interna
      b. tunica media
      c. tunica externa

C. Cardiac
   1. Right heart
   2. Left heart

D. Coronary Blood Flow
   1. Left anterior descending
   2. Circumflex
   3. Right coronary artery
   4. Collateral circulation

E. Movement of Blood
   1. Systole
      a. contraction of atria and ventricles
   2. Diastole
      a. filling of the atria and ventricles
      b. filling of the coronary arteries
   3. Contractile filaments
      a. actin
      b. myosin
   4. Muscle stretch
   5. Muscle strength
   6. Preload

IV.   Cellular Physiology

A. Myocardial Cells
1. Resting cell membrane
   a. sodium outside
   b. calcium outside
   c. potassium inside
2. Action potential

B. Electrical Cells
1. Electrical stimulation
2. Actin
3. Myosin
4. Intercalated discs
5. Automaticity
6. Conductivity

V.   Electrical System

A. Sinoatrial Node

B. Atrioventricular Node

C. Interatrial Pathways
1. Bachmann's bundle

D. Internodal Pathways

E. AV Junction

F. Bundle of His

G. Bundle Branches

H. Purkinje Fibers

I. Myocardial "Working Cells"

VI. Normal Cardiac Cycle

A. P Wave - Atrial Depolarization

B. QRS - Ventricular Depolarization

C. T Wave - Ventricular Repolarization

D. P-R Interval - AV Node Delay

E. S-T Segment - Completion of QRS to Onset of Repolarization

VII. Autonomic Nervous System

A. Influence on Heart Rate, Conductivity, Strength and Force

B. Cardiac Output

C. Divisions
   1. Sympathetic
   2. Parasympathetic

D. Medications
   1. Chronotropic
   2. Inotropic

VOCABULARY

Action potential
Autonomic
Cardiac output
Chronotropic
Collateral circulation
Conductivity
Contractility
Depolarization
Diastole
Inotropic
Myocardium
Parasympathetic
Preload
Repolarization
Stroke volume
Sympathetic
Systole

REVIEW QUESTIONS

◊ What is the approximate size of a normal adult heart?

◊ Why is the heart considered to be a "double pump"?

◊ What information does the ECG tracing provide about the condition of the heart?

◊ Which portion of the autonomic nervous system is often described as eliciting the "fight or flight" response?

◊ What is the name of the innermost layer in arteries and veins?

◊ Which two electrolytes are found outside of the cell membrane when the myocardial cell is completely repolarized?

◊ What is the purpose of the intercalated discs?

◊ What is the name of the valve located between the left atrium and ventricle?

◊ Which heart valves close during the S-1 heart sound?

◊ Which heart valves close during the S-2 heart sound?

◊ Which ECG waveform represents ventricular repolarization?

◊ Which portions of the heart are considered to be supraventricular?

◊ What is the action of an inotropic medication?

◊ What is the purpose of the fluid normally found inside the pericardial sac?

◊ What is the relationship between diastole and preload?

PATHOPHYSIOLOGY OF CORONARY ARTERY DISEASE

GOALS

After completing this lesson the student will be able to demonstrate knowledge of:

◊ common causes of coronary artery disease.

◊ the risk factors associated with coronary artery disease.

◊ the specific areas of the electrical conduction system and myocardium supplied by each coronary artery.

◊ the events that often precipitate angina or myocardial infarction.

◊ the effects of diminished blood flow on the myocardium.

◊ the importance of early recognition and intervention of coronary artery disease.

◊ the mechanism of collateral circulation.

◊ the incidence of sudden death associated with myocardial infarction.

◊ the difference between stable angina, unstable angina and acute myocardial infarction.

◊ the difference between transmural and non-transmural infarction.

◊ the signs and symptoms associated with angina.

◊ the major complication associated with myocardial infarction.

◊ the treatment modalities of thrombolytic therapy and beta blockade.

OBJECTIVES

◊ List the five types of angina.

◊ Discuss the insidious nature of coronary artery disease.

◊ Describe the progression of atherosclerosis within the coronary arteries.

◊ Identify risk factors that increase the propensity for coronary artery disease.

◊ Describe how decreased blood flow to the myocardium may be detected on the ECG tracing.

◊ Recognize the incidence of dysrhythmias associated with myocardial infarction.

◊ Explain the effects of hypertension and tachycardia on myocardial oxygen consumption.

◊ Discuss the significance of angina that occurs at rest.

◊ Discuss the mechanism of collateral circulation as it applies to coronary artery disease.

◊ Discuss the significance of chest pain that is not relieved by the administration of nitroglycerin.

◊ Describe what occurs when a ventricle ruptures.

◊ Explain the mechanism of coronary vasospasm.

◊ Correlate the effects of a thromboembolism as it applies to each of the coronary arteries.

◊ Name the location of the heart most susceptible to infarction.

OUTLINE

I. **Introduction**

    A. Pathophysiology of Coronary Artery Disease

    B. Angina

    C. Myocardial Infarction
       1. Complications

II. **Coronary Artery Disease**

    A. Atherosclerosis
       1. Incidence
       2. Onset
       3. Progression
       4. Collateral circulation
       5. Ischemia
       6. Angina

    B. Thromboembolism
       1. Location
          a. left main coronary artery
          b. left anterior descending artery
          c. circumflex artery
          d. right coronary artery

III. **Angina Pectoris**

    A. Myocardial Ischemia

    B. Precipitating Events

    C. Onset While Resting

    D. Signs and Symptoms

E. Chronic Stable Angina
  1. Predictable
  2. Transient
  3. Recurrent pattern
  4. Fixed narrowing of coronary arteries
  5. Advanced atherosclerosis

F. Unstable Angina
  1. Abrupt change in pain
  2. Crescendo angina
  3. Severe coronary artery obstruction

G. Variant Angina (Prinzmetal's)
  1. Onset at rest
  2. Coronary artery spasm
  3. Atypical ECG tracing
  4. Cyclic pattern

H. Intractable Angina
  1. Unresponsive to treatment

I. Postinfarction angina
  1. onset after myocardial infarction

J. Complications of Angina
  1. Ventricular dysrhythmias
  2. Left ventricular failure
  3. Myocardial infarction
  4. Psychological depression

IV. Complications of Acute Myocardial Infarction

A. Etiology
  1. Thrombus
  2. Coronary artery spasm
  3. Decreased blood supply
     a. atherosclerotic narrowing
     b. shock
     c. dysrhythmias
     d. pulmonary embolism

B. Tissue Necrosis

C. Location
   1. Left ventricle
      a. inferior wall
      b. anterior wall
      c. anterolateral wall
      d. anteroseptal
   2. Right ventricle

D. Types of Infarction
   1. Subendocardial
   2. Transmural

E. Contributing Factors
   1. Extent of infarct
      a. vessel involved
      b. collateral circulation
   2. Myocardial oxygen consumption
      a. hypertension
      b. tachycardia
   3. Onset
      a. rest
      b. moderate activity

F. Signs and Symptoms
   1. Substernal pain
   2. Unrelieved by nitroglycerin
   3. Associated signs and symptoms

G. "Silent MI"

H. Complications
   1. Cardiogenic shock
      a. inadequate tissue perfusion
      b. heart failure

   2. Dysrhythmias
      a. ninety per cent incidence
      b. typically ventricular
      c. frequent cause of sudden death

   3. Thromboembolism
      a. source
      b. common locations

   4. Rupture left ventricle
      a. weakened ventricular wall
      b. pericardial tamponade
      c. typically 7-10 days post MI
      d. high mortality rate

I. Treatment
   1. Early recognition and intervention
   2. Thrombolytic therapy
   3. Beta blockers

VOCABULARY

Atherosclerosis
Arteriosclerosis
Asymptomatic
Ischemia
Necrosis
Precipitating
Thrombolytic
Thrombosis
Transmural

REVIEW QUESTIONS

◊ Why is the occurrence of angina at rest considered a serious sign of heart disease?

◊ What are the five types of angina?

◊ What is the most common cause of coronary artery disease?

◊ What are some common risk factors that may increase the incidence and severity of coronary artery disease?

◊ Why is coronary artery disease considered to be an insidious disease?

◊ What is a "silent MI"?

◊ In what way is the administration of nitroglycerin used to differentiate angina from a myocardial infarction?

◊ Occlusion of which coronary artery typically results in the most extensive myocardial damage?

◊ Which ECG rhythm often results in sudden death?

◊ Why does infarction occur more commonly in the left ventricle?

◊ What conditions can increase the oxygen consumption of the myocardium?

◊ Which two medications are often administered for the treatment of a myocardial infarction?

◊ What are some common locations for the formation of emboli?

◊ Why is collateral circulation beneficial in the presence of a myocardial infarction?

ECG Monitoring

GOALS

After completing this lesson the student will be able to demonstrate knowledge of:

◊ electrophysiology.

◊ the conduction system.

◊ principles of depolarization, repolarization and refractoriness.

◊ proper electrode placement and patient preparation.

◊ graphic indicators on ECG paper.

◊ techniques of calculating heart rate.

◊ the five step method for evaluating cardiac rhythms.

◊ the criteria for normal ECG waveforms and P,Q,R,S,T relationships.

◊ basic physical assessment of cardiac patients.

OBJECTIVES

◊ Use the five step rhythm method to interpret normal ECG rhythms.

◊ Describe the relationship between the heart's conduction system and the ECG waveform.

◊ State the location and function of the sinoatrial and atrioventricular nodes.

◊ Name and define the two types of cardiac cells.

◊ Define the phases of systole and diastole as they relate to blood flow through the cardiac chambers.

◊ State the inherent rates of the SA node, AV node and ventricles.

◊ Label the P,Q,R,S,T components of a normal complex.

◊ Differentiate between electrical and mechanical activity.

◊ Demonstrate electrode placement of leads I, II, III and MCL1.

◊ Use several methods to calculate heart rate.

◊ Discuss how heart rate can affect a patient's physical status.

◊ Recognize which ECG waveforms yield information about atrial conduction.

◊ Recognize which ECG waveforms yield information about ventricular conduction.

OUTLINE

I. Electrical Conduction System

A. Conductivity

B. Cardiac Cells
  1. Electrical
     a. automaticity
  2. Working
     a. contractility

C. Pathways
  1. Sinoatrial
  2. Internodal
  3. Interatrial
  4. Atrioventricular
  5. Bundle of His
  6. Purkinje network

D. Pacemakers
  1. Sinoatrial
  2. Escape pacemakers
     a. AV junction
     b. Ventricles
  3. Automatic rates

II. ECG Waveforms

A. Atrial Depolarization
  1. P-wave

B. Ventricular Depolarization
　　1. QRS complex

C. Atrial Repolarization
　　1. Buried within QRS complex

D. Ventricular Repolarization
　　1. T wave
　　2. Refractory period

III. Mechanical Function

A. Cardiac Output
　　1. Pulse, blood pressure
　　2. Mental status

IV. Electrodes

A. Patient Preparation

B. Placement

V. Leads

A. Deflections
　　1. Positive
　　2. Negative
　　3. Bipolar
　　4. Ground
　　5. Isoelectric

B. Specific Leads
　　1. Leads I through III
　　2. Limb leads
　　3. Modified chest leads

VI. Five Step Rhythm Analysis

    A. Rate
    B. Rhythm
    C. QRS duration*
    D. Atrial Activity
    E. P to QRS Relationship

VII. ECG Tracings

    A. Graph Paper
        1. Time intervals
        2. Amplitude
        3. Duration

    B. Heart Rate Calculation
        1. Six second method
        2. ECG calipers
        3. 300, 150, 100 method

    C. Rhythm

VIII. Specific Sinus Rhythms

    A. Normal Sinus Rhythm

    B. Sinus Bradycardia

    C. Sinus Tachycardia

    D. Sinus Arrhythmia

    E. Sinus Arrest

*note: Most ECG texts recognize .10 seconds as a normal QRS duration. Others state that any QRS less than .12 seconds is acceptable. A general rule to follow is that any QRS complex wider than .12 seconds indicates conduction below the AV junction.

VOCABULARY

Amplitude
Automatic rate
Automaticity
Bipolar
Bradycardia
Complex
Cycle
Diastole
Escape
Ground
Isoelectric
MCL
Refractory
Tachycardia
Voltage

REVIEW QUESTIONS

◊ What is the automatic rate of the SA node, AV node and ventricles?

◊ What is the duration of a normal QRS complex?

◊ What is the duration of a normal P - R interval?

◊ What attempts can be made to improve electrode contact on a patient?

◊ The P-R interval indicates a delay in which portion of the cardiac conduction system?

◊ Why is there not a waveform that indicates repolarization of the atria?

◊ What length of time is indicated by five large boxes on the ECG paper?

◊ In what sequence do the atria and ventricles normally contract?

◊ What are the components of the five step rhythm analysis method?

◊ The pulse should correspond with which waveform?

◊ What are the electrode positions for leads I, II, III and MCL1?

◊ What rhythm may result when an impulse is initiated during the relative refractory period of the T-wave?

◊ What signs and symptoms might be displayed by a patient with a sinus bradycardia?

◊ How can respirations affect the regularity of the heart?

CASE STUDIES

1. Mrs. Wilson is 64 years old. She is complaining of general weakness, shortness of breath and chest pain since awakening this morning. Vital signs are: pulse156 and regular, respirations 20, BP 144/80.

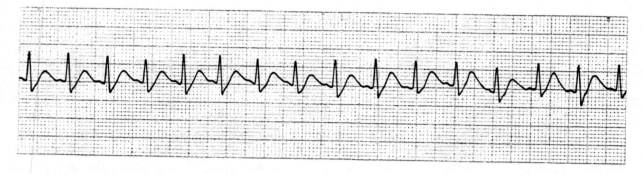

2. Jack is a 23 year-old triathlete. He is being evaluated for his annual physical exam. Vital signs are: pulse 52, respirations 14, BP 110/60.

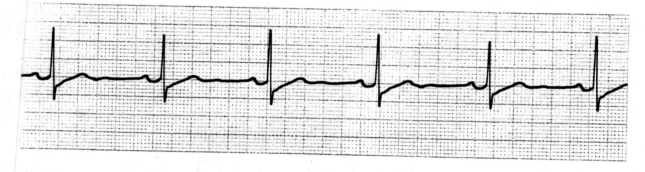

3. 12 year-old Sally is a patient in your pediatric unit recovering from an emergency appendectomy. You note that her pulse is slightly irregular and place her on the ECG monitor for further evaluation. Vital signs are: pulse 66, respirations 16, BP 100/50.

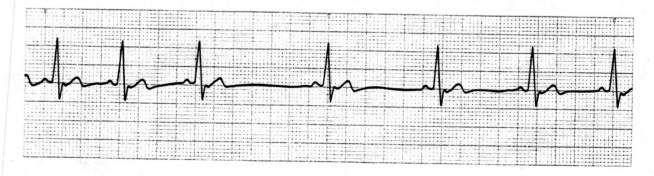

4. Mr. Mullins is a 45 year-old corporate executive seeking treatment in the emergency department today for abdominal pain. His vital signs are: pulse 72 and regular, respirations 18, BP 136/70. As part of your assessment you place him on the ECG monitor.

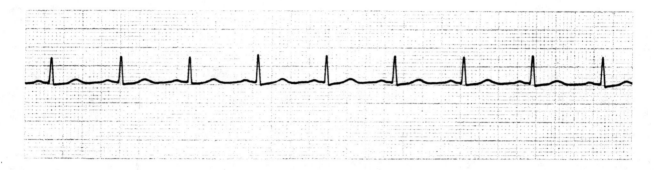

GOALS

After completing this lesson the student will be able to demonstrate knowledge of:

◊ the pathways of electrical conduction within the atria.

◊ the concept of "atrial kick".

◊ abnormal impulse formation.

◊ normal and aberrant ventricular conduction.

◊ AV nodal reentry mechanisms.

◊ the mechanism of triggered activity.

◊ the potential effects of altered automaticity.

◊ the effect of tachycardia on coronary artery perfusion.

◊ the determination of stable and unstable atrial rhythms.

◊ the therapeutic modalities of drug therapy, vagal maneuvers and synchronized cardioversion.

◊ the clinical implications of atrial dysrhythmias with rapid ventricular response rates.

OBJECTIVES

◊ Use the five step rhythm method to interpret atrial dysrhythmias.

◊ Describe the phases of systole and diastole as they apply to coronary artery perfusion.

◊ Discuss the importance of determining atrial and ventricular rates.

◊ List and define the three types of abnormal impulse formation.

◊ Explain normal and aberrant conduction of premature atrial contractions.

◊ Recognize cardiovascular and pulmonary conditions that can occur in patients with sustained tachycardia.

◊ Differentiate between atrial fibrillation, flutter and tachycardia.

◊ List three medications used for conversion of atrial dysrhythmias with rapid ventricular rates.

◊ Recognize atrial rhythms that may require synchronized cardioversion.

◊ Demonstrate techniques for applying vagal maneuvers.

◊ Describe the potential hemodynamic effects of acute, unstable atrial tachydysrhythmias.

OUTLINE

I. Introduction

    A. Review of Five Step Rhythm Analysis Method
        1. Rate
        2. Rhythm
        3. QRS duration
        4. Atrial activity
        5. P to QRS relationship

    B. Causes of Atrial Dysrhythmias
        1. Ischemia or myocardial infarction
        2. Electrolyte imbalances
        3. Cardiac diseases
        4. Altered autonomic regulation
        5. Non-therapeutic ranges of drug levels

II. Atrial Function

    A. Collection Chambers

    B. "Atrial Kick"

III. Atrial Conduction

    A. Sinoatrial Node

    B. Intra-atrial Pathways
        1. Bachmann's bundle

    C. AV node

    D. Working Cells
        1. Conductivity
        2. Excitability

IV. Abnormal Impulse Formation

A. Triggered Activity

B. Altered Automaticity

C. Reentry

V. Premature Atrial Complex

A. Criteria
1. P-wave configuration
2. P to QRS relationship
3. Rhythm - noncompensatory pause
4. QRS width

B. Conduction
1. Normal
2. Aberrant
3. Nonconducted

C. Mechanism
1. Ectopic focus
2. Digitalis
3. Electrolyte imbalance
4. Stimulants

D. Clinical Significance
1. Usually none

E. Treatment
1. Remove stimulants
2. Evaluate digitalis levels

VI. Atrial Tachycardia

A. Criteria
   1. Rate, rhythm and duration of QRS
   2. Atrial activity

B. Mechanism
   1. Triggered activity
   2. Altered automaticity
   3. Reentry

C. Hemodynamic Implications
   1. Coronary artery blood flow
   2. Ventricular filling time
   3. Sytemic tissue perfusion
   4. Myocardial oxygen consumption

D. Clinical Significance
   1. Rate related
   2. Diminished cardiac output

E. Paroxysmal Atrial Tachycardia
   1. Criteria

F. Therapeutic Modalities
   1. Vagal maneuvers
   2. Synchronized cardioversion
   3. Medications
   4. Overdrive pacing

VII. Multiformed Atrial Rhythms

A. Criteria
   1. Rate rhythm and duration of QR
   2. P-wave configurations
   3. P to QRS relationship

B. Mechanism
    1. Triggered activity

C. Clinical Significance
    1. Good prognosis <100 per minute
    2. Poor prognosis   >100 per minute

D. Treatment
    1. Assess and manage underlying cause

VIII. Atrial Flutter

A. Criteria
    1. Rate, rhythm and QRS duration
    2. F waves
    3. Conduction ratios and degree of block
    4. Flutter to R-wave relationship

B. Mechanism
    1. Single reentry circuit
    2. Ischemic heart disease

C. Clinical Significance
    1. Related to ventricular rate
    2. Loss of atrial kick

D. Treatment Modalities
    1. Medications
    2. Synchronized cardioversion
    3. Vagal stimulation

IX. Atrial Fibrillation

A. Criteria
    1. Rate, rhythm and duration of QRS
    2. Fib wave to QRS relationship
    3. Atrial activity

B. Mechanism
1. One or more ectopic foci
2. Mitral valve disease
3. Ischemic heart disease

C. Clinical Significance
1. Rate related
2. Systemic embolization
3. Heart failure

D. Treatment
1. Anticoagulation
2. Medications
3. Synchronized cardioversion
4. Vagal stimulation

X. **Wolff-Parkinson-White Syndrome**

A. Criteria
1. Rate, rhythm and duration of QRS
2. Delta wave
3. P to QRS relationship
4. T-wave changes

B. Mechanism
1. Genetic disease
2. Accessory pathways
3. Preexcitation

C. Clinical Significance
1. Diminished cardiac output
2. Potential shock

D. Differentiation from Ventricular Tachycardia
1. WPW irregular
2. V-Tach usually regular

    E. Treatment
        1. Vagal stimulation
        2. Medications
        3. Transcutaneous pacing

XI. Supraventricular Tachycardia

    A. Definition

    B. Patient Tolerance
        1. Stable
        2. Unstable

XII. Patient Assessment

    A. Tolerance of Ventricular Rate
        1. Hemodynamic compromise >150 per minute
        2. Vital signs
        3. End organ perfusion
        4. Medical history
        5. Subjective complaints

XIII. Treatment Modalities

    A. Vagal Maneuvers
    B. Synchronized cardioversion

VOCABULARY

Aberrant
Accessory pathway
Altered automaticity
Altered autonomic regulation
Atrial kick
Controlled
Ectopic
Focus
Hemodynamic
Hypertrophy
Infarction
Paroxysmal
Reentry
Supraventricular
Synchronize
Thromboembolism
Transcutaneous
Transvenous
Triggered Activity
Uncontrolled
Vagal

REVIEW QUESTIONS

◊ What is an ectopic focus?

◊ What percentage of blood flow is contributed by the "atrial kick"?

◊ How would you define reentry?

◊ At greater than what heart rate do multiformed atrial rhythms have a poor prognosis?

◊ How would you describe the difference between fibrillatory and flutter waves?

◊ Which signs and symptoms would you expect to observe in a patient with an atrial flutter rhythm with a ventricular response of 170/min.?

◊ What is meant by noncompensatory pause?

◊ How would you identify an aberrantly conducted beat?

◊ What effects do tachycardic rhythms have on coronary artery blood flow and ventricular filling time?

◊ What are the three categories of drugs for treating atrial dysrhythmias?

◊ When applying synchronized cardioversion, upon which ECG waveform does the monitor deliver the shock?

◊ Which cranial nerve is stimulated by applying carotid sinus massage?

◊ Why is it important to determine if a patient is stable or unstable?

◊ What is the purpose of anticoagulant therapy prior to cardioversion?

CASE STUDIES

1. Anna is a 20 year-old nursing student studying all night for final exams. She has had 5 cups of coffee and 12 cigarettes over the past 4 hours. She arrives at your emergency department complaining of chest palpitations and numbness in her hands and face. Her vital signs are: pulse 80, respirations 44, BP 128/80. Her ECG shows:

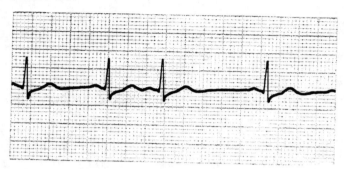

2. A 67 year-old male arrives via ambulance in your emergency department. His history includes a myocardial infarction one year ago and frequent episodes of angina. Today he is complaining of palpitations, nausea and dyspnea. He appears restless and agitated. His skin is pale, cool and clammy. His vital signs are: pulse 160, respirations 30 and shallow, BP 84/66.

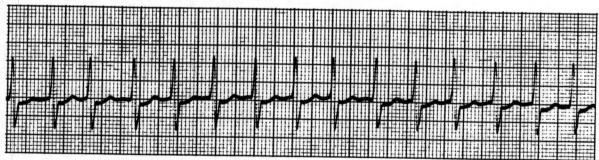

3. 83 year-old Mrs. Gifford is brought code 3 to the emergency department for an altered level of consciousness. She has a 20 year history of diabetes and COPD. Vital signs are: pulse 122, respirations assisted at 20 per minute, BP 90/68. The ECG monitor shows:

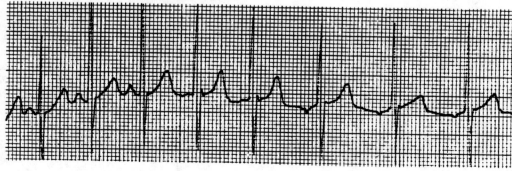

4.   Mrs. Thompson is a 70 year-old female in your clinic for a routine blood draw to check her cholesterol and digitalis levels. She has a history of congestive heart failure. She has no complaint of pain or signs of peripheral edema and states that she has been healthy and relatively active for the past two months. Pulse is 68 and irregular, respirations 20, BP 152/80.

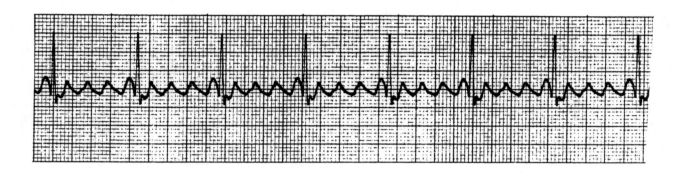

5.   Mr. Edwards is a 60 year-old retired police officer admitted to your ICU for treatment of right lobar pneumonia. His vital signs are: pulse 168, respirations 26, BP 140/90. He complains of moderate chest pain upon deep inspiration.

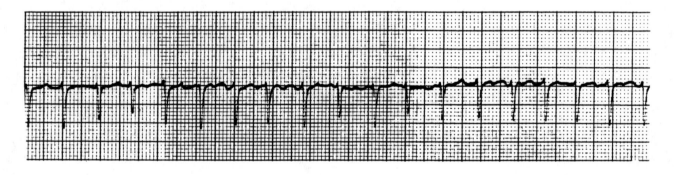

6. An ambulance is called to transport a 17 year-old female high school student who has experienced two syncopal episodes while sitting in Spanish class. School officials suspect a drug overdose. Paramedics obtain vital signs of: rapid and weak peripheral pulse (unable to count rate), respirations 26 and shallow, BP 90/48. She is oriented to name and age only. Her skin is pale, cool and moist with delayed capillary refill. Her ECG shows:

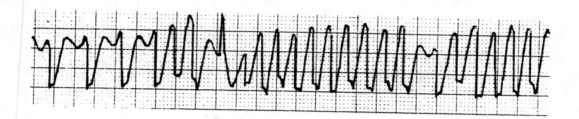

7. While sitting at the telemetry console, you notice that Mr. Sandoval's ECG rhythm suddenly changes from a regular sinus rhythm to the rhythm below:

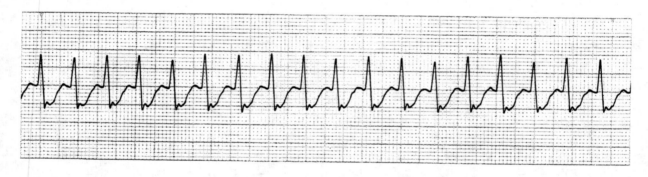

Upon your appropriate treatment his rhythm is now:

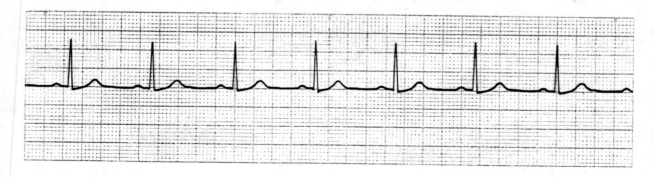

JUNCTIONAL DYSRHYTHMIAS

GOALS

After completing this lesson the student will be able to demonstrate knowledge of:

◊ the three zones of the AV junction.

◊ the concept of escape pacemakers.

◊ the mechanism of altered automaticity.

◊ the clinical implications of slow and tachycardic junctional rhythms.

◊ the therapeutic modalities of drug therapy, vagal maneuvers, transcutaneous pacing, overdrive pacing and synchronized cardioversion.

◊ anterograde and retrograde conduction as it applies to P wave morphology.

◊ normal and aberrant ventricular conduction.

◊ the incidence of digitalis toxicity in junctional dysrhythmias.

OBJECTIVES

◊ Use the five step rhythm method to analyze junctional dysrhythmias.

◊ State common causes of junctional dysrhythmias.

◊ Correlate P wave morphology and P-R intervals with origin and speed of conduction within the AV junction.

◊ Discuss the principles of escape mechanism as they relate to junctional dysrhythmias.

◊ Describe the hemodynamic consequences of asynchronous beating of the heart.

◊ Differentiate between accelerated and tachycardic junctional rhythms.

◊ Identify normal and aberrant ventricular conduction associated with junctional dysrhythmias.

◊ Recognize the importance of checking digitalis levels in the presence of junctional dysrhythmias.

◊ Understand the goals for treating symptomatic junctional tachycardias.

◊ List the indications for the electrical therapies of transcutaneous pacing, transvenous pacing, synchronized cardioversion, overdrive pacing and vagal maneuvers used in the treatment of junctional rhythms.

◊ Define the term supraventricular tachycardia as it applies to junctional dysrhythmias.

◊ Explain the relationship between lead selection and P wave direction.

OUTLINE

I. Introduction

A. Review of Five Step Rhythm Analysis Method
1. Rate, rhythm and duration of QRS
2. Atrial activity
3. P to QRS relationship

II. Divisions of the AV Junction

A. Conduction Zones
1. Upper region - transitional - slow conduction
2. Middle region - middle - rapid conduction
3. Lower region - His bundle - rapid conduction

B. Back-up Pacemaker

III. Junctional P Waves

A. Retrograde Conduction
1. Speed of impulse
2. Origin of impulse

B. P Wave Morphology
1. Inverted
2. Short P-R interval
3. Hidden
4. After QRS complex

IV. Junctional QRS Complexes

A. Normal Ventricular Conduction

B. Aberrant Ventricular Conduction

V. Premature Junctional Complexes

A. Criteria
1. QRS rate, rhythm and duration
2. Early atrial activity
3. P to QRS relationship

B. Mechanism
1. Ectopic focus
2. Ischemic heart disease
3. Digoxin toxicity

C. Clinical Significance
1. Usually none
2. Possible digitalis toxicity

D. Treatment
1. Eliminate stress and stimulants
2. Evaluate digitalis levels

VI. Junctional Escape Rhythm

A. Criteria
1. QRS rate, rhythm and duration
2. Atrial activity
3. Early, hidden or late P to QRS relationship
4. Sinus pause

B. Mechanism
1. Failure of SA node
2. Hyperkalemia
3. Medications

C. Clinical Significance
1. Potential signs and symptoms of hypoperfusion

D. Treatment
1. Medications
2. Temporary or permanent pacing

VII. Accelerated Junctional Rhythm

   A. Criteria
      1. Rate, rhythm and duration of QRS
      2. Atrial activity
      3. Early, hidden or late P to QRS relationship
      4. Gradual or paroxysmal onset

   B. Mechanism
      1. Altered automaticity or triggered activity
      2. Inflammatory disease of the heart
      3. COPD
      4. Digitalis toxicity

   C. Clinical Significance
      1. Usually none
      2. Loss of "atrial kick"

   D. Treatment
      1. Close monitoring
      2. Evaluate digitalis level

VIII. Junctional Tachycardia

   A. Criteria
      1. Rate, rhythm and duration of QRS
      2. Atrial activity
      3. Early, hidden or late P to QRS relationship
      4. Gradual or paroxysmal onset

   B. Mechanism
      1. Altered automaticity or triggered activity
      2. Acute myocardial infarction

   C. Clinical Significance
      1. Improper AV synchrony
         a. cannon waves
      2. Congestive heart failure
      3. Digitalis toxicity
      4. Potential signs and symptoms of hypoperfusion

D. Treatment
1. Medications
2. Evaluate digitalis levels
3. Vagal maneuvers
4. Synchronized cardioversion
5. Overdrive pacing

IX. Patient Management

A. Hypoperfusion
1. Related to ventricular rate
   a. too slow
   b. too fast
2. Patient tolerance

B. Objective Signs of Symptomatic Tachycardia
1. Altered level of consciousness
2. Dyspnea
3. Poor skin perfusion
4. Inadequate urine output
5. Pulmonary edema
6. Peripheral edema
7. Cannon waves

C. Subjective Signs
1. Weakness
2. Palpitations
3. Chest pain
4. Shortness of breath

D. Medications
1. Calcium channel blockers
2. Beta blockers
3. Digitalis
4. Adenosine
5. Atropine
6. Isoproterenol
7. Quinidine
8. Catecholamines

E. Vagal Maneuvers
   1. Instruct patient to Valsalva
   2. Diver's reflex
   3. Carotid sinus massage

F. Synchronized Cardioversion
   1. Indicated for unstable patients
   2. Heart rates typically >150 per minute
   3. Depolarization timed with the R wave
   4. Application techniques
   5. Safety

G. Transcutaneous External Pacing
   1. Indicated for symptomatic bradycardia
   2. Demand mode
   3. Electrode placement
      a. anterior-anterior
      b. anterior-posterior
   4. Safety
   5. Rate
   6. Intensity
   7. Capture

H. Overdrive Pacing
   1. Indicated for symptomatic tachycardia
   2. Trained personnel only

I. Other Treatment Modalities
   1. Remove stimulants
   2. Evaluate digitalis level
   3. Evaluate electrolyte levels
   4. Insure adequate oxygenation and ventilation

VOCABULARY

Anterograde
Cannon waves
Capture
Demand
Joules
Milliamps
Retrograde
Symptomatic
Threshold

REVIEW QUESTIONS

◊ What is the rate range for accelerated junctional rhythm?

◊ What is the difference between altered automaticity and an escape mechanism?

◊ Where is the origin of impulse if the P-R interval is less than 0.12 seconds?

◊ What are the pathways of conduction for a retrograde P wave?

◊ How would you explain the inversion of the P wave in junctional rhythms?

◊ How is aberrant ventricular conduction different from normal conduction?

◊ When applying synchronized cardioversion, upon which ECG waveform does the monitor deliver the shock?

◊ In what way are transcutaneous and transvenous pacing different?

◊ Why is it important to determine how well a patient is tolerating a junctional escape rhythm?

◊ What signs and symptoms would you expect to observe if a patient presented with a junctional tachycardia at 170 per minute?

◊ Which medications can be given to convert junctional tachycardia?

◊ Which medications can be given to treat junctional escape rhythm?

◊ What instructions can be given to a conscious and cooperative patient to stimulate the vagus nerve?

CASE STUDIES

1. Arthur is a 36 year-old asthma patient in your clinic for a refill of theophylline. He states that he occasionally experiences a "missed beat." His vital signs are within normal limits. As a precaution you place him on the ECG monitor.

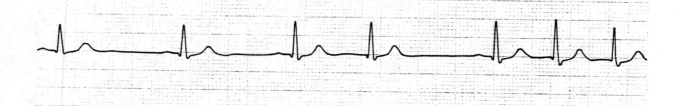

2. Mrs. Davenport is a 62 year-old woman recently released from the hospital after treatment for myocarditis. She is in today for a follow-up exam. Vital signs are: pulse 160, respirations 18, BP 104/70. The ECG shows:

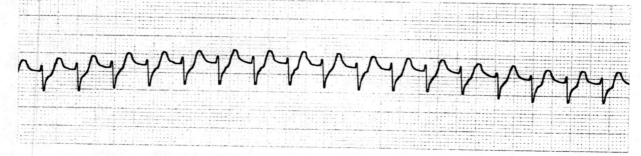

3. Mr. Chung is a 54 year-old man brought in to the emergency department by his wife. He is complaining of severe substernal chest pain and dyspnea that started three hours ago while grocery shopping. Vital signs are: pulse 40 and weak, respirations 30 and shallow, BP 78/40. Skin signs are pale, cool and moist with delayed capillary refill. His ECG reveals:

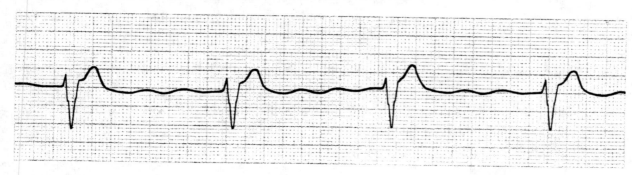

VENTRICULAR DYSRHYTHMIAS

GOALS

After completing this lesson the student will be able to demonstrate knowledge of:

◊ conduction within the ventricles.

◊ the principles of single and multiple foci.

◊ the terminology used to describe ventricular dysrhythmias.

◊ the factors contributing to myocardial irritability.

◊ the mechanisms of altered automaticity, reentry and escape.

◊ the morphology of ventricular dysrhythmias.

◊ the potentially lethal nature of ventricular dysrhythmias.

◊ the clinical implications of ventricular dysrhythmias.

◊ the therapeutic modalities of drug and electrical therapy.

◊ the criteria for determining stable versus unstable patients with ventricular dysrhythmias.

OBJECTIVES

◊ Use the five step rhythm analysis method to analyze ventricular dysrhythmias.

◊ Differentiate between unifocal and multifocal ventricular ectopy.

◊ Define the criteria for the compensatory pause associated with most premature ventricular complexes.

◊ Discuss the basis of the morphology of ventricular dysrhythmias.

◊ List five sources of ventricular irritability.

◊ Discuss the lethal nature of ventricular tachycardia, fibrillation and standstill.

◊ Discuss cardiac output and the hemodynamic consequences of ventricular dysrhythmias.

◊ Recognize R on T phenomenon and its effect on repolarization.

◊ Identify specific ventricular dysrhythmias caused by reentry, altered automaticity and escape mechanisms.

◊ Describe how you would assess the relationship of electrical impulses and the mechanical response of the myocardium.

◊ Demonstrate the therapeutic modalities of synchronized cardioversion and defibrillation.

◊ List three medications that are classified as antiarrhythmic.

◊ List specific criteria for deciding when to treat ventricular ectopy.

◊ Discuss the value of oxygen therapy in managing patients with ventricular dysrhythmias.

OUTLINE

I. Introduction

   A. Review of Five Step Rhythm Analysis Method
      1. Rate
      2. Rhythm
      3. QRS duration
      4. Atrial activity
      5. P to QRS relationship

II. Structures and Function of the Ventricles

   A. Bundle Branches

   B. Purkinje Network

   C. Ventricles
      1. Right
      2. Left
      3. Automatic rate

III. Premature Ventricular Complexes

   A. Criteria
      1. QRS rate, rhythm and duration
      2. Atrial activity
      3. P to QRS relationship
      4. T wave
      5. Compensatory pause
      6. Interpolated
      7. R on T phenomenon
      8. Unifocal
      9. Multifocal
     10. Patterns

B. Mechanism
   1. Altered automaticity or reentry
   2. Ischemia or infarction
   3. Structural or inflammatory disease
   4. Electrolyte imbalances
   5. Adrenergic stimulation

C. Clinical Significance
   1. Related to frequency
   2. Sign of cardiac irritability

D. Treatment Criteria
   1. Frequency
   2. Focus
   3. Pattern
   4. Associated signs and symptoms
   5. Potential for R on T

E. Treatment
   1. Oxygen
   2. Remove stressors
   3. Medications

IV. **Ventricular Tachycardia**

A. Criteria
   1. Rate, rhythm and duration of the QRS
   2. Atrial activity
   3. P to QRS relationship
   4. Three or more consecutive PVCs

B. Mechanism
   1. Altered automaticity or reentry
   2. Ischemia or infarction
   3. Acid-base imbalance
   4. R on T phenomenon
   5. Hypokalemia

C. Clinical Significance
  1. With pulses
      a. stable
      b. unstable
  2. Without pulses
  3. Lethal rhythm

D. Treatment - With Pulses
  1. Antiarrhythmic medications
  2. Synchronized cardioversion

E. Treatment - Without Pulses
  1. Defibrillation
  2. Basic life supprt
  3. Antiarrhythmic medications

V. Torsades de Pointes

A. Criteria
  1. Rate, rhythm and duration of QRS
  2. Atrial activity
  3. P to QRS relationship
  4. Morphology

B. Mechanism
  1. Electrolyte imbalances
  2. Acute ischemia
  3. Reaction to antiarrhythmic medications

C. Clinical Significance
  1. Lethal rhythm

D. Treatment
  1. Magnesium sulfate
  2. Isoproterenol
  3. Synchronized cardioversion

VI. Ventricular Fibrillation

A. Criteria
 1. Unorganized chaotic activity
 2. Fine versus coarse

B. Mechanism
 1. Refractory to ventricular tachycardia
 2. Ischemia or infarction

C. Clinical Significance
 1. Complete circulatory collapse

D. Treatment
 1. Confirm rhythm
 2. Defibrillate
 3. Basic life supprt
 4. Antiarrhythmic medications

VII. Ventricular Escape

A. Criteria
 1. Rate, rhythm and duration of QRS
 2. Atrial activity
 3. P to QRS relationship

B. Mechanism
 1. Backup pacemaker
 2. SA or AV nodal disease
 3. Heart blocks

C. Clinical Significance
 1. Bradycardia
 2. Decreased cardiac output and hypoperfusion

D. Treatment
    1. Assess tolerance
    2. Medications to increase rate
    3. Transcutaneous or transvenous pacemaker
    4. Basic life support

VIII. Ventricular Asystole

A. Criteria
    1. No ventricular activity
    2. Possible atrial activity

B. Mechanism
    1. Significant myocardial damage
    2. Post termination of tachydysrhythmias

C. Clinical Significance
    1. Complete circulatory collapse

D. Treatment
    1. Confirm rhythm
    2. Basic life support
    3. Transcutaneous pacing
    4. Medications

VOCABULARY

Antiarrhythmic
Bigeminy
Couplet
Dissociation
Inherent
Interpolated
Multifocal
Quadrigeminy
Trigeminy
Unifocal
Viability

REVIEW QUESTIONS

◊ Why are the majority of ventricular rhythms considered serious?

◊ What rhythm may occur when an impulse is initiated during ventricular repolarization?

◊ What is another term for ventricular standstill?

◊ Which ventricular rhythms can result from an irritable myocardium?

◊ What is the difference between ventricular escape and multiple PVCs?

◊ Why do most PVCs have a compensatory pause?

◊ Why are multifocal PVCs considered more serious than unifocal PVCs?

◊ Which three antiarrhythmic drugs are typically administered for ventricular fibrillation?

◊ What effect does defibrillation have on the myocardial cells?

◊ Why is synchronized cardioversion only appropriate when a patient has a pulse?

◊ Why would it be lethal to administer lidocaine to a ventricular escape rhythm?

◊ How can oxygen therapy affect myocardial irritability?

◊ When would it be necessary to insert a permanent transvenous pacemaker?

◊ What is the differentiating characteristic between ventricular tachycardia and torsades de pointes?

CASE STUDIES

1. Yvonne is a 41 year-old billing clerk in the emergency department. You notice that she looks pale today and convince her to allow you to assess her further. Her vital signs are: pulse 88 and irregular, respirations 24, BP 100/54. Upon placing her on the ECG monitor you see:

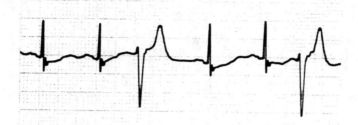

2. You are bedside in the step down unit assisting Mr. Foster with his dinner when he complains of an acute onset of chest pain. Glancing at the monitor you see the rhythm below. Vital signs are: pulse 160 and weak, respirations 24, BP 88/40.

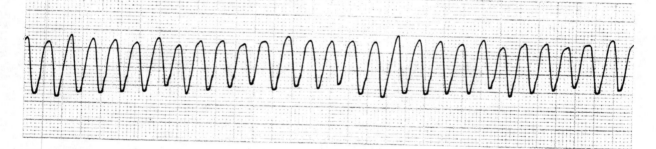

Five minutes have passed after initiating treatment for Mr. Foster. His vitals are now: absent pulse, no spontaneous respiratory effort, no blood pressure.The monitor shows:

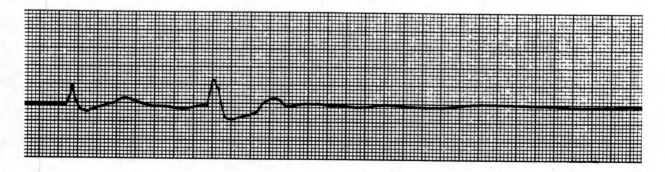

3. An unconscious 22 year-old female is brought by ambulance to the emergency department. Her family found a suicide note and an empty bottle of her grandmother's quinidine pills nearby. Paramedics initiated CPR two minutes prior to arrival at your facility. The ECG monitor shows:

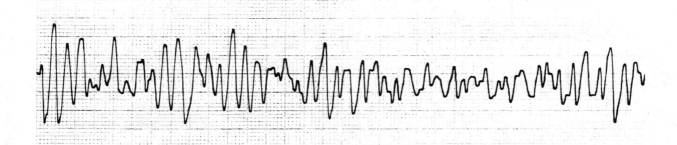

4. You respond via rescue squad to a manufacturing plant where a 38 year-old man has received a 6,000 volt shock from a power transformer. He is pulseless and apneic. The ECG monitor shows:

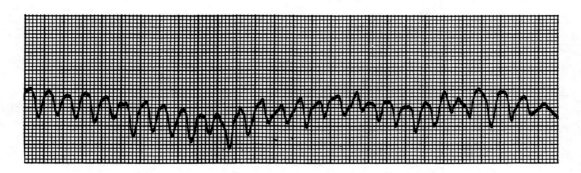

5. Mr. Lang is a 70 year-old man admitted to the ICU this afternoon after a bypass of his right coronary artery. Currently he is complaining of dizziness, general weakness and nausea. His vital signs are: pulse 36 and weak, respirations 26 and labored, BP 78/46. His ECG monitor shows:

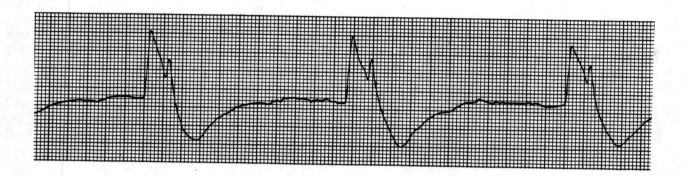

The ICU staff have been working on Mr. Lang for approximately fifteen minutes. He is now pulseless and respirations are being assisted via bag valve mask with 100% oxygen. His rhythm is now:

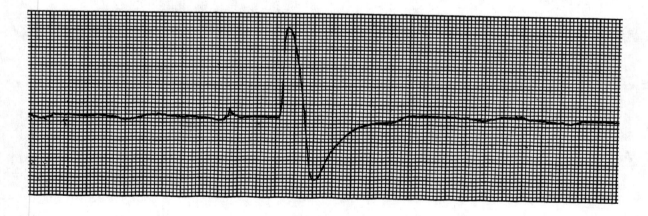

AV HEART BLOCKS

GOALS

After completing this lesson the student will be able to demonstrate knowledge of:

◊ the importance of the P to QRS relationship in AV blocks.

◊ the location and degrees of AV blocks.

◊ the prognosis of the four types of AV blocks.

◊ delayed, partial and completely blocked conduction.

◊ factors contributing to AV blocks.

◊ medications that enhance AV node conduction.

◊ the indications for transcutaneous and transvenous pacing.

◊ the clinical significance of each type of AV block.

◊ the origin of escape rhythms associated with complete heart block.

◊ AV blocks resulting from insufficient right or left coronary artery blood flow.

◊ junctional and ventricular escape rhythms associated with third degree AV block.

OBJECTIVES

◊ Apply the five step rhythm method to interpret AV heart blocks.

◊ Differentiate between partial and complete AV blocks.

◊ Discuss the principles of delayed conduction.

◊ Explain the significance of prolonged P-R intervals.

◊ Determine the location of an AV block based on the degree of blocked conduction.

◊ Recognize the relationship between ventricular response rate and cardiac output.

◊ State which AV blocks have a fixed P-R interval.

◊ State which AV blocks have a regular ventricular rhythm.

◊ List the indications for pacemaker therapy as a treatment for AV block.

◊ Describe the clinical presentation of a patient with symptomatic second degree type II or third degree heart block.

◊ List two medications that improve conduction through the AV node.

◊ Define the term AV dissociation.

◊ Explain the significance of non-conducted P waves.

◊ Describe the difference between junctional and ventricular escape rhythms as they apply to AV blocks.

◊ Discuss the difference between right and left coronary blood flow as it applies to AV heart blocks.

OUTLINE

I. Introduction

    A. Five Step Rhythm Analysis Method
1. Rate
2. Rhythm
3. QRS duration
4. Atrial activity
5. P to QRS relationship

II. Categories of AV Blocks

    A. Slowed Conduction
1. First degree block

    B. Partially Blocked Conduction
1. Second degree block - type I
2. Second degree block - type II

    C. Complete Block
1. Third degree block

III. First Degree AV Block

    A. Criteria
1. Rate, rhythm and duration of QRS
2. Atrial activity
3. P to QRS relationship

    B. Mechanism
1. Ischemia or infarction
2. Medications that slow AV conduction
3. Increased parasympathetic tone
4. Right coronary artery disease

    C. Clinical Significance
1. Usually none

D. Treatment
1. Rate dependent
2. Evaluate current drug levels

IV. Second Degree Block - Type I (Wenckebach)

A. Criteria
1. Rate, rhythm and duration of QRS
2. Atrial activity
3. P to QRS relationship
4. Dropped complexes

B. Mechanism
1. AV nodal block
2. Ischemia or infarction
3. Right coronary artery disease
4. Post open heart surgery
5. Increased parasympathetic tone
6. Electrolyte imbalance

C. Clinical Significance
1. Often transient
2. Rate dependent

D. Treatment
1. Monitor for further block
2. Assess hemodynamic status
3. Evaluate current drug levels
4. Evaluate serum electrolytes
5. Medications
6. Transcutaneous pacing

V. Second Degree Block - Type II (Mobitz Type II)

A. Criteria
1. Rate, rhythm and duration of QRS
2. Atrial activity
3. P to QRS relationship
4. Dropped complexes

B. Mechanism
   1. Infranodal block
   2. Ischemia or infarction
   3. Left coronary artery disease
   4. Cardiomyopathy

C. Clinical Significance
   1. Usually permanent block
   2. Rate dependent

D. Treatment
   1. Assess hemodynamic status
   2. Medications
   3. Transcutaneous or transvenous pacemaker

VI. Third Degree Block

A. Criteria
   1. Rate, rhythm and duration of QRS
   2. Atrial activity
   3. Atrial rate
   4. P to QRS complex
   5. Junctional escape
   6. Ventricular escape

B. Mechanism
   1. Complete AV nodal or bundle block
   2. Ischemia or infarction
   3. Left coronary artery disease
   4. Sclerotic heart disease

C. Clinical Significance
   1. Usually permanent block
   2. Rate dependent

D. Treatment
   1. Assess hemodynamic status
   2. Medications
   3. Transcutaneous or transvenous pacemaker

VII. Patient Assessment

A. Stable Versus Unstable

B. Assessment Parameters

VIII. Treatment Modalities

A. Evaluate Potential Causative Drugs
1. Digitalis
2. Beta blockers
3. Calcium channel blockers
4. Quinidine

B. Medications
1. Atropine
2. Epinephrine
3. Dopamine
4. Isoproterenol

C. Electrical Therapy
1. Transcutaneous pacing
2. Transvenous pacing
3. Placement
4. Intensity
5. Rate
6. Pain management
7. Troubleshooting
8. Demand versus fixed mode
9. Safety
10. Documentation

VOCABULARY

Infranodal
Mobitz
Nodal
Wenckebach

REVIEW QUESTIONS

◊ Which two types of AV block can be caused by insufficient blood flow through the right coronary artery?

◊ Which two types of AV block can be caused by insufficient blood flow through the left coronary artery?

◊ What is the predominant difference between second degree AV blocks type I and II?

◊ In third degree block, which escape rhythm has a better prognosis?

◊ Why is it important to measure both atrial and ventricular rates?

◊ What is meant by the term "demand" mode pacing?

◊ What signs and symptoms would you expect in a patient with an AV block with a ventricular rate of 30 beats per minute?

◊ What are some common medications that can be responsible for the slowed AV conduction associated with some heart blocks?

◊ What are some important assessment parameters for evaluating a patient's tolerance to an AV block?

◊ How can ischemic and necrotic tissue affect electrical conduction?

◊ Why is an infranodal block more severe than a nodal block?

◊ Which two types of AV blocks have fixed P-R intervals?

◊ Which two types of AV blocks have an irregular ventricular response?

◊ When is it appropriate to apply a temporary or permanent pacemaker?

CASE STUDIES

1. Mr. Katz is a 63 year-old man receiving a routine dialysis treatment. His medications are digitalis, procardia and furosemide. The nurse notes that his pulse is 54 and decides to place him on the ECG monitor for further evaluation. He denies any pain or distress. Respirations 18, BP 122/78.

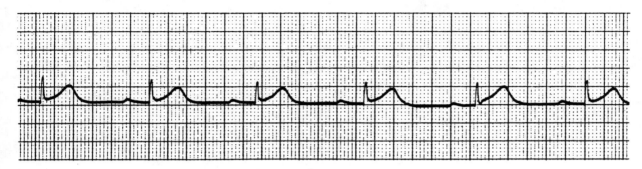

2. Rachel is a 34 year-old woman transferred to your ICU post mitral valve surgery. Six hours after the surgery she is resting quietly with stable vital signs. On the monitor you see:

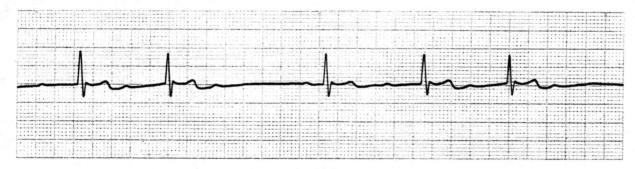

3. Mrs. Sterling is a 71 year-old obese woman stating that she is having difficulty tolerating the hot weather this summer. She complains of chronic fatigue, general malaise and occasional "fainting spells." She is pale, cool and slightly moist. Vital signs are: pulse 40, respirations 22, BP 80/44.

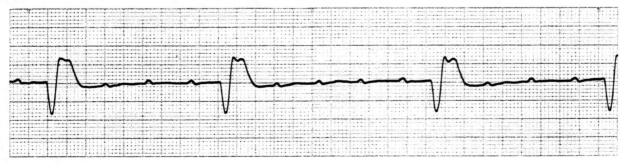

4. Paramedics are called to a convalescent home to find a 76 year-old man complaining of general weakness and nausea. Facility staff states he was unable to walk to the dining room for breakfast this morning. He has a history of a stroke and two previous MIs. A pacemaker can be palpated under his right clavicle. The ECG monitor shows:

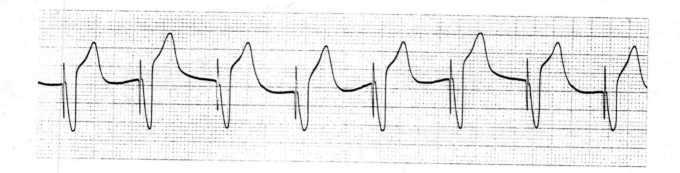

5. Albert is a 59 year-old postal carrier who collapsed on the sidewalk while delivering the mail. A passerby found him confused and unable to sit up. Paramedics placed him on the ECG monitor and obtained vital signs of: pulse 32 and weak, respirations 26, BP 76/48. His skin is pale, cool and diaphoretic with peripheral cyanosis and delayed capillary refill.

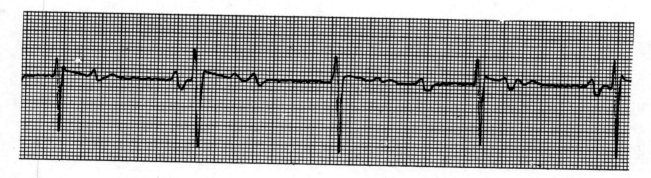

12- LEAD ECG

GOALS

After completing this lesson the student will be able to demonstrate knowledge of:

◊ the 12-lead perspective of cardiac conduction.

◊ normal magnitude and direction of electrical vectors.

◊ the criteria for axis determination.

◊ causes of abnormal axis deviation.

◊ normal waveform configuration in each lead.

◊ Einthoven's triangle and law for calculation of the zero potential reference point.

◊ the hexaxial reference system.

◊ correct lead placement for 12-lead ECG analysis.

◊ 12-lead determination of intraventricular conduction blocks.

◊ common 12-lead changes associated with pericarditis.

◊ the leads associated with frontal and horizontal planes of the heart.

◊ normal R wave progression.

◊ coronary artery blood supply to the conduction system.

◊ adverse drug effects indicated on the 12-lead ECG.

OBJECTIVES

◊ Compare unipolar, bipolar and precordial leads.

◊ State the degree designations and rotation of the hexaxial reference system.

◊ Calculate an electrical axis using the hexaxial reference system.

◊ Discuss intraventricular conduction defects of the bundle of His and its branches.

◊ Correlate the coronary arteries with each component of the cardiac conduction system.

◊ Differentiate between anterior and posterior hemiblocks.

◊ State the normal polarity and morphology of the P,Q,R,S,T waveforms in each of the 12 leads.

◊ State why the unipolar leads require augmentation.

◊ Demonstrate proper placement of the precordial leads.

◊ Discuss the stages of septal and ventricular activation as it applies to the 12-lead ECG.

◊ Understand the relationship between digitalis and potassium blood levels.

◊ Describe 12-lead ECG changes commonly associated with digitalis toxicity.

◊ State the sequence of normal R wave progression.

◊ State common 12-lead features for diagnosing pericarditis.

OUTLINE

I.   Introduction

   A. Electrical Activity
       1. Positive pole
       2. Negative pole

   B. Planes
       1. Frontal
       2. Horizontal

II. Leads

   A. Limb Leads
       1. Placement of leads I, II and III
       2. Bipolar
       3. Frontal plane
       4. Einthoven's triangle

   B. Augmented Leads
       1. Placement of AVR, AVL and AVF
       2. Unipolar
       3. Low amplitude
       4. Frontal plane

   C. Precordial Leads
       1. Placement of V1 - V6
       2. Horizontal plane

III. Normal 12-lead Configurations

   A. Vectors
       1. Magnitude
       2. Direction
       3. Depolarization
       4. Positive ECG deflection

B. Activation
   1. Septal and initial right ventricle
   2. Right and left ventricular wall
   3. Mean QRS vector - left

C. Depolarization
   1. Toward positive electrode
   2. Away from positive electrode
   3. Perpendicular with positive electrode

D. P Wave
   1. Atrial depolarization
   2. Direction
   3. Width
   4. Height

E. QRS Complex
   1. Ventricular depolarization
   2. Direction
   3. Width
   4. Height

F. R Wave
   1. Septal depolarization
   2. V-1 direction
   3. Width
   4. Height

G. Q Wave
   1. Septal depolarization
   2. V-6 direction
   3. Width
   4. Height

H. R Wave Progression
   1. Increasing from V-1 to V-6

IV. Electrical Axis

A. Hexaxial Reference System
1. Frontal - most equiphasic or isoelectric QRS
2. Perpendicular - largest QRS complex
3. Degree designations
4. Positive pole
5. Negative pole

B. Axis
1. Normal range
2. Left axis deviation
3. Right axis deviation
4. "Northwest quadrant", "No man's land"

V. Intraventricular Conduction Defects

A. Structures of Electrical Conduction System
1. Bundle of His
2. Right bundle branch
3. Left bundle branch
   a. left anterior fascicle
   b. left posterior fascicle

B. Blood Supply to Electrical Conduction System
1. Right coronary artery
   a. AV node
   b. bundle of His
   c. left posterior division
2. Left anterior descending artery
   a. right bundle branch
   b. left anterior fascicle
   c. left posterior fascicle

C. Bundle Branch Activation
1. Normal
2. Blocked
3. Common causes of blocked conduction

    D. Right Bundle Branch Block
        1. QRS >0.12 seconds
        2. Positive QRS in lead V-1
        3. R, S, R' in lead V-1
        4. ST depression and T wave inversion in leads V-1 and V-2

    E. Left Bundle Branch Block
        1. QRS >0.12 seconds
        2. Negative QRS in lead V-1
        3. rS or QS configuration
        4. Wide R wave in leads V-5 and V-6
        5. Absent septal Q waves in leads V-5, V-6, I and AVL

VI. Pericarditis

    A. Pathophysiology

    B. 12-lead Changes
        1. Diffuse ST elevation
        2. T wave inversion

VII. Medications

    A. 12-lead Changes Associated with Digitalis
        1. Downward sloping ST segment
        2. Flattened or inverted T wave
        3. Slowed AV conduction

    B. Digitalis Toxicity
        1. Ventricular dysrhythmias
        2. AV block
        3. Tachycardia
        4. Potentiated by hypokalemia

C. Quinidine
1. Slowed conduction
2. Wide, notched P wave
3. Wide QRS
4. Prolonged QT interval
5. Depressed ST segment
6. Potential for Torsades de Pointes

VOCABULARY

Activation
Augment
Diphasic
Equiphasic
Fascicle
Hexaxial
Intraventricular
"No man's land"
"Northwest quadrant"
Perpendicular lead
Plane
Polarity
Precordial
Prime
Unipolar
Vector

REVIEW QUESTIONS

◊ What do vectors indicate?

◊ Which coronary artery supplies the posterior division of the left bundle branch?

◊ Why are the standard limb leads considered bipolar?

◊ Which leads divide the heart into top and bottom halves?

◊ Which electrolyte imbalance can potentiate digitalis toxicity?

◊ What are some common causes of abnormal axis deviation?

◊ What are the names of the two divisions of the left bundle branch?

◊ How does ventricular activation occur when a conduction block is located in a bundle branch?

◊ During which leads should normal R wave transition occur?

◊ Why do the unipolar limb leads require augmentation?

◊ How can improper electrode placement alter the ECG tracing?

◊ Which ECG waveform indicates normal septal activation?

◊ Why is it important to find the most equiphasic QRS complex when determining the axis of the heart?

◊ What do the terms "northwest quadrant" and "no man's land" refer to?

◊ Which disease can cause ST segment elevation not associated with myocardial injury?

CASE STUDIES

1. Rhonda is 29 years old. She is 8 months pregnant and being seen in the out-patient clinic today for hypertension, headaches and generalized edema. Vital signs are: pulse 90, respirations 20, BP 148/96. Her 12-lead ECG rhythm shows:

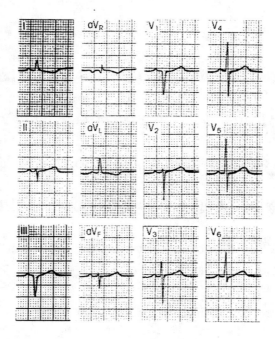

2. Mr. Zigler is a 66 year-old retired air force pilot admitted to your ICU
last night for an acute pulmonary embolism. A 12-lead ECG is ordered with
morning labs. Vital signs are: pulse 90, respirations 32, BP 112/80.
His 12-lead ECG shows:

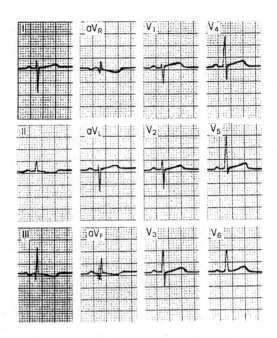

3. Mrs. Flaherty is a 56 year-old high school swim coach required to have a 12-lead ECG test as part of an insurance examination. She is active and healthy. Her family history includes cardiovascular disease on both sides of the family. To date she has had no cardiac related health problems. Her ECG shows:

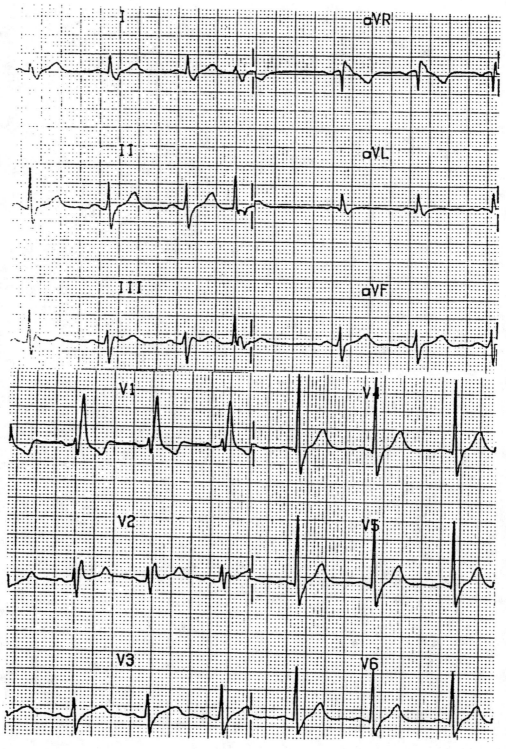

4. Mrs. Klein is a 68 year-old woman with chronic heart problems. She recently moved to the area and was referred to your facility for a complete physical examination. She states that she has had two previous myocardial infarctions within the past four years. Her vital signs are within normal limits. The 12-lead ECG shows:

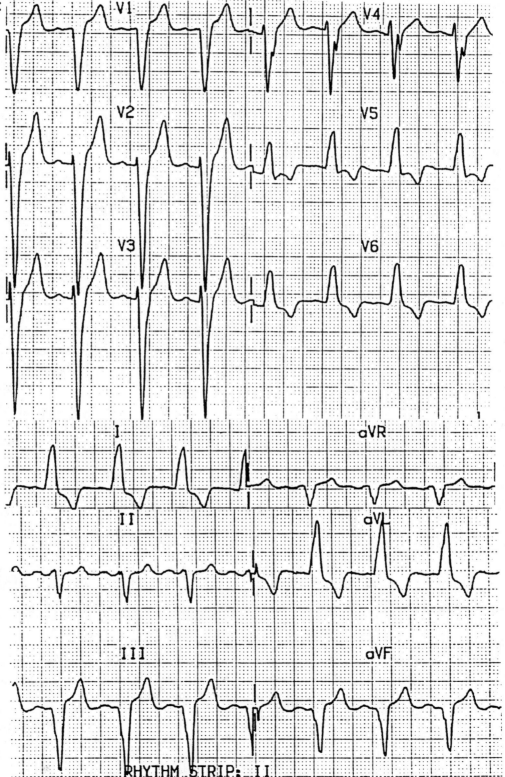

5. Mr. Overton is a 71 year-old male visting your clinic this morning for a routine check-up. While his blood is being drawn to check his cholesterol and digitalis levels, he states that he has been having difficulty concentrating lately. He also complains of yellowing vision and an increased sensitivity to sunlight. His vital signs are normal for his age. The 12-lead ECG shows:

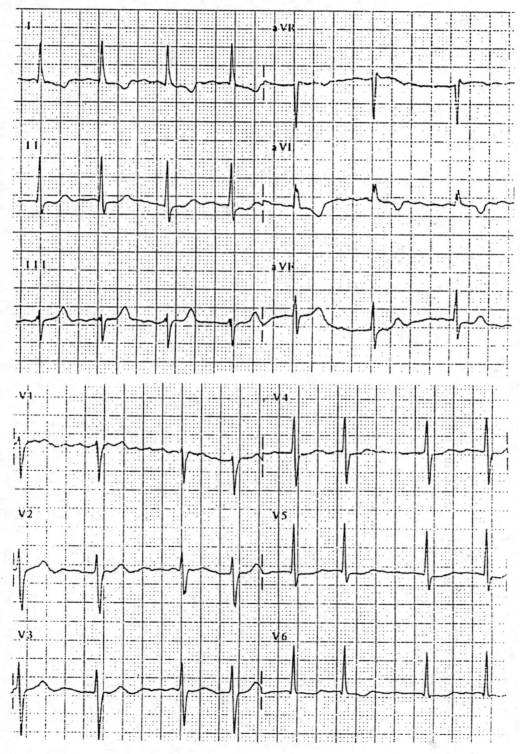

ISCHEMIA, INJURY AND INFARCTION

GOALS

After completing this lesson the student will be able to demonstrate knowledge of:

◊ the pathophysiology of an acute myocardial infarction.

◊ sources of increased myocardial oxygen consumption.

◊ common 12-lead ECG changes associated with injury, ischemia or infarction of the myocardium.

◊ specific complications associated with occlusion of the right, left and circumflex coronary arteries.

◊ the concept of dominance as it applies to myocardial blood supply.

◊ the effects of atherosclerosis on myocardial blood supply.

◊ 12-lead ECG changes indicative of Prinzmetal's angina.

◊ the sequence of ECG changes in an evolving myocardial infarction.

◊ the value of CK-MB isoenzyme testing.

◊ clinical signs and symptoms of right and left sided heart failure.

◊ the indications and contraindications for thrombolytic therapy.

◊ situations in which myocardial damage may be reversible.

◊ the morphology of pathological Q waves.

◊ the implications of ST segment elevation.

OBJECTIVES

◊ Explain the basic pathophysiology of a myocardial infarction.

◊ Recognize the need for early intervention in patients presenting with signs of myocardial damage.

◊ State the difference between myocardial ischemia, injury and infarction.

◊ Correlate the 12-lead ECG changes associated with an evolving myocardial infarction.

◊ Discuss the mechanism of a non-Q wave myocardial infarction.

◊ Explain the importance of evaluating CK-MB isoenzyme levels in the differential diagnosis of a myocardial infarction.

◊ Describe why the course of treatment differs for left- and right-sided myocardial infarctions.

◊ List the criteria that qualify a patient for thrombolytic therapy.

◊ Discuss the incidence of sudden death and life threatening dysrhythmias associated with myocardial infarction.

◊ State the method for diagnosing a posterior wall infarction.

◊ Correlate each lead as it relates to specific locations of the heart.

◊ Discuss the difficulties encountered in diagnosing an infarction when a left bundle branch block is present.

◊ Describe the clinical differences between left- and right-sided heart failure.

◊ Discuss the importance of evaluating the ST segment.

OUTLINE

I. **Introduction**

    A. Incidence of Myocardial Infarction

    B. Definition of Myocardial Infarction

    C. Importance of Recognition

    D. Application of 12-lead Interpretation

    E. Criteria for Thrombolytic Therapy

II. **Pathophysiology**

    A. Blood Supply to the Myocardium
        1. Origin of coronary arteries
        2. Systole
        3. Diastole

    B. Right Coronary Artery
        1. Location
        2. Structures supplied
        3. Right dominance

    C. Left Coronary Artery
        1. Location
        2. Structures supplied
        3. Left dominance

    D. Circumflex Branch
        1. Location
        2. Structures supplied

    E. Atherosclerosis

    F. Myocardial Oxygen Consumption

III. Ischemia, Injury and Infarction

A. Progression

B. Ischemia
1. Inverted T waves
2. ST depression

C. Injury
1. ST elevation >1mm

D. Prinzmetal's Angina
1. Variant
2. ST elevation without infarction

E. Infarction
1. Pathologic Q waves >.04 seconds wide
2. Q waves greater than one third the QRS
3. Old versus new infarcts
4. Reciprocal changes
5. Sequence of ECG changes
    a. increase in T wave amplitude
    b. ST elevation
    c. pathological Q waves
    d. diminished R wave amplitude
    e. T wave inversion

IV. Infarct Location

A. Incidence of Left Ventricular Infarct

B. Anterior Wall
1. Leads V-1 through V-4

C. Lateral Wall
1. V-5, V-6, I and AVL

    D. Inferior Wall
        1. Leads II, III and AVF

    E. Posterior Wall
        1. Reciprocal changes in leads V-1 through V-4
        2. Often associated with inferior wall infarct

    F. 12-lead Changes Indicating Infarction

    G. Infarction in the Presence of Left Bundle Branch Block

V. Other Indicators of Myocardial Infarction

    A. Clinical Signs and Symptoms
        1. Chest pain unrelieved by nitroglycerin

    B. Creatine Kinase-Myocardial Band Isoenzyme Levels
        1. Peak ~24 to 36 hours after infarction

    C. Non-Q Wave Myocardial Infarction

VI. Complications Associated with Myocardial Infarction

    A. Anterior Wall Infarction
        1. Pump failure
        2. Atrial or ventricular dysrhythmias
        3. Intraventricular conduction disturbances

    B. Inferior Wall Infarction
        1. Pump failure
        2. Bradydysrhythmias
        3. Second degree AV block type I (Wenckebach)

    C. Posterior Wall Infarction
        1. Signs and symptoms similar to inferior wall infarction
        2. Dysrhythmias involving the SA node, AV node and His bundle

VII. Right Ventricular Infarction

A. Right Chest Precordial Lead Placement

B. ST Segment Elevation >1mm in V-4, V-5 and V-6.

C. Potential for AV Block

D. Treatment
   1. Caution with diuretics and vasoactive agents
   2. Maintain adequate cardiac output
      a. volume expansion to increase preload
      b. vasodilators
      c. inotropic agents

VIII. Thrombolytic Therapy

A. Goals
   1. Provide for acute needs
      a. high flow oxygen
      b. pain management
      c. cardiovascular support
      d. treat life threatening dysrhythmias
   2. Assess qualification for thrombolytic therapy
      a. chest pain <6 hours unrelieved by nitroglycerin
      b. ST elevation in multiple leads
      c. under 75 years old

B. Pharmacologic Effects
   1. Reperfusion by dissolving of thrombi or clots

VOCABULARY

Dominance
Infarction
Injury
Pathologic
Reciprocal

REVIEW QUESTIONS

◊ Which leads indicate an inferior wall MI?

◊ Which leads indicate an anterior wall MI?

◊ Why is early intervention important in the treatment of MI?

◊ What condition is indicated by a "tombstone" T wave?

◊ What are some common causes of increased myocardial oxygen consumption?

◊ Which component of the ECG complex offers the most information about the oxygenation of the myocardium?

◊ How can you identify an evolving MI based on ECG changes?

◊ In which ventricle does a myocardial infarction most commonly occur?

◊ How would you differentiate an old from a new infarction?

◊ In addition to coronary artery occlusion, what conditions may also cause an elevated ST segment?

◊ What occurs within the myocardium to cause a pathologic Q wave?

◊ What are the two primary goals for thrombolytic therapy?

◊ What criteria qualify a patient for thrombolytic therapy?

◊ What method is used to determine a right-sided myocardial infarction?

◊ Approximately how many hours does it take for CK-MB isoenzymes to reach peak levels?

CASE STUDIES

1. Mr. Mathern is a 48 year-old attorney admitted to your ICU for treatment and observation one day after being diagnosed with a myocardial infarction. He is currently pain-free with stable vital signs. You obtain a copy of his last 12-lead ECG to determine the area of myocardial damage.

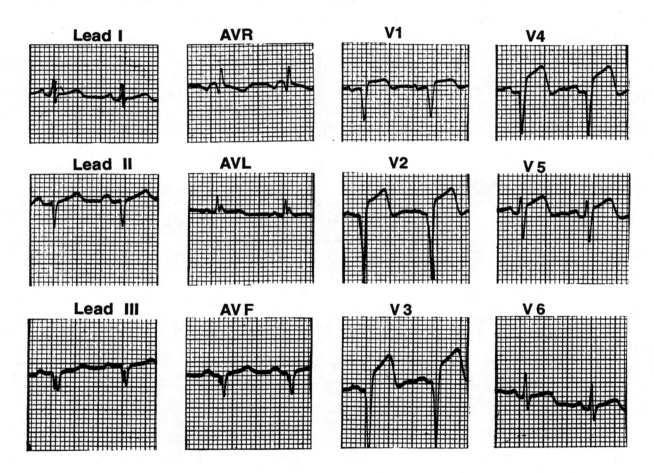

2. Mr. Micelli is a 59 year-old overweight gourmet chef. He is brought to your emergency department via paramedic ambulance with complaints of severe substernal non-radiating chest pain that began one hour ago. He experiences no relief from sublingual nitroglycerin or six liters of oxygen by nasal cannula. He is pale, cool and diaphoretic with weak peripheral pulses. Upon physical assessment you observe moderate jugular vein distention and +1 pitting pedal edema. His vital signs are: pulse 54, respirations 26 with fine scattered crackles, BP 152/94. The medical student is bedside with the 12-lead ECG and asks your opinion about the area of infarct.

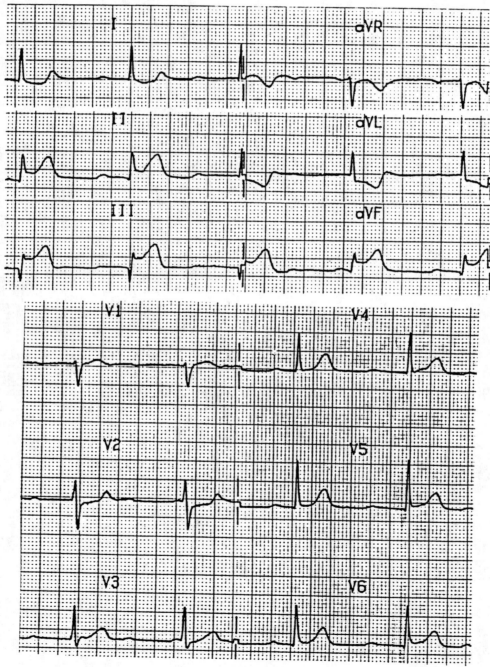

3. Mrs Quesada is a 60 year-old homemaker in your telemetry unit 3 days after being diagnosed with a posterior wall infarction. She is pain-free with stable vital signs. The telemetry technician pulls the 12-lead ECG out of her chart and asks you to show him the 12-lead changes that indicate a posterior wall infarction.

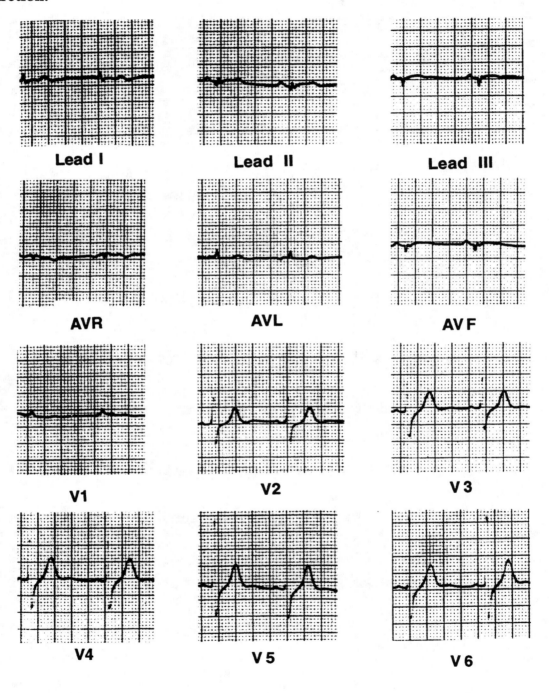

Lead I Lead II Lead III

AVR AVL AVF

V1 V2 V3

V4 V5 V6

DIFFERENTIAL INTERPRETATION

GOALS

After completing this lesson the student will be able to demonstrate knowledge of:

◊ the importance of history and physical exam in diffential diagnosis.

◊ the 12-lead ECG differences between ventricular tachycardia and supraventricular tachycardia with aberrancy.

◊ the 12-lead ECG differences between block acceleration dissociation and complete third degree AV block.

◊ the 12-lead ECG differences between Torsades de Pointes and ventricular fibrillation.

◊ the technique of diagnosis by exclusion.

◊ the significance of QRS morphology in diagnosing ventricular tachycardia.

◊ common etiologies of Torsades de Pointes.

◊ therapeutic interventions for the treatment of Torsades de Pointes.

◊ the differences in treatment for ventricular tachycardia and supraventricular tachycardia with aberrancy.

◊ the importance of determining a relationship between atrial and ventricular activity.

OBJECTIVES

◊ Discuss the significance of QRS morphology when differentiating ventricular tachycardia from supraventricular tachycardia with aberrancy.

◊ State the statistical incidence of ventricular tachycardia versus supraventricular tachycardia.

◊ Recognize the importance of determining an association between atrial and ventricular activity.

◊ State the differences between block acceleration dissociation and third degree AV block.

◊ Describe the relationship between prolonged QT intervals and Torsades de Pointes.

◊ State two common treatments for Torsades de Pointes.

◊ Discuss the significance of evaluating the polarity of the QRS complexes in the precordial leads when diagnosing ventricular tachycardia.

◊ Recognize the importance of a complete history and physical examination as they relate to differential diagnosis.

◊ Name the two leads that are the most beneficial in the differential interpretation of wide complex tachycardias.

◊ State three techniques for stimulating the vagus nerve.

OUTLINE

I. Introduction

    A. Differential Diagnosis
        1. Ventricular tachycardia
        2. Supraventricular tachycardia
        3. Block acceleration dissociation
        4. Torsades de Pointes

    B. When to Treat
        1. History and physical indicators
        2. ECG interpretation

    C. How to Treat
        1. Monitor
        2. Medications
        3. Electrical therapy
        4. Vagal maneuvers

II. Wide Complex Tachycardias

    A. Axis Determination
        1. Leads I, II and III

    B. QRS Morphology in Ventricular Tachycardia
        1. Taller left rabbit ear in MCL1 or V-1
        2. Negative complex with R wave >.04 seconds
        3. Negative QS complex without initial R wave in MCL6 or V-6
        4. QRS >.14 seconds

    C. QRS Morphology in SVT with Aberration
        1. Triphasic in MCL1 or V-1
        2. Triphasic in MCL6 or V-6
        3. Ectopic atrial activity prior to onset
        4. Comparison of pre-existing bundle branch block
        5. Response to vagal stimulation, medication and cardioversion

    D. Step by Step 12-lead ECG Evaluation
        1. Precordial leads
        2. P wave association
        3. QRS morphology

III. Block Acceleration Dissociation

    A. Common Misdiagnosis of Third Degree AV Block

    B. Undetermined Degree of AV Block

    C. AV Dissociation
        1. Source of accelerated pacemaker
        2. Rate of pacemaker

    D. Associated History and Symptoms

IV. Torsades de Pointes

    A. Multiformed QRS Complexes

    B. Refractory Period
        1. Prolonged QT interval
        2. Delayed repolarization of ventricles

    C. Etiologies

    D. Treatment
        1. Medications
        2. Overdrive pacing

VOCABULARY

Differential
Exclusion
"Rabbit ears"
"Tombstone" T waves
Triphasic

REVIEW QUESTIONS

◊ Which wide complex tachycardia is indicated when the QRS complex is >.14 seconds wide?

◊ Which wide complex tachycardia is more prevalent, ventricular tachycardia or supraventricular tachycardia with aberrancy?

◊ How does the morphology of Torsades de Pointes differ from ventricular tachycardia?

◊ Why is it helpful to observe the onset of a wide complex tachycardia?

◊ What is the purpose of evaluating the P waves when differentiating block acceleration dissociation from third degree AV block?

◊ Why is ventricular rate an important factor in diagnosing block acceleration dissociation?

◊ What might happen if ventricular tachyardia were treated with verapamil?

◊ By what mechanism does isoproterenol treat Torsades de Pointes?

◊ What are some of the important assessment parameters in the differential diagnosis of wide complex tachycardia and block acceleration dissociation rhythms?

◊ Why is QRS morphology a critical component of differential diagnosis?

◊ Which portion of the QRS "rabbit ears" become elevated in the presence of ventricular tachycardia?

◊ Which axis will always be displayed by ventricular tachycardia?

CASE STUDIES

1. Mr. Petersen is a 68 year-old retired fisherman staying in your medical ICU after a massive anterior MI. You are bedside administering a scheduled medication when he becomes unresponsive. His skin appears ashen and peripheral pulses are barely palpable. The bedside monitor shows a wide complex tachycardia. His vital signs are: pulse 160, respirations 28, BP 90/50. A stat 12-lead ECG is ordered.

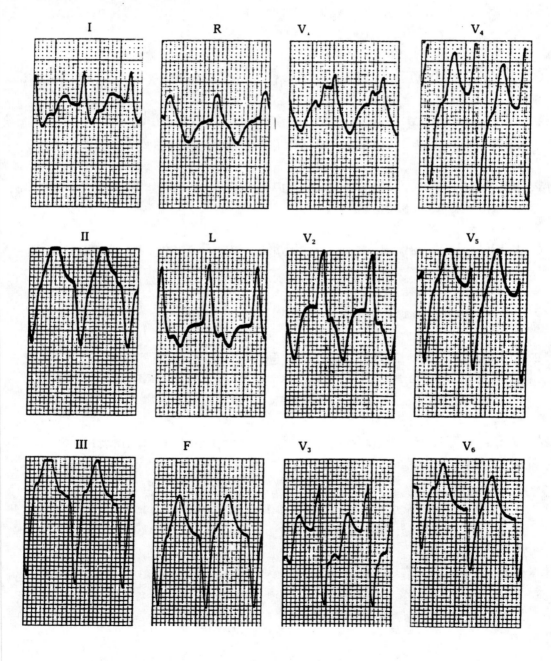

2. Mrs. Pietro is a 59 year-old florist seeking treatment in the emergency
   department for recurrent episodes of fluttering in her chest. She state she feels
   weak and nauseated during the episodes that typically last three to five minutes.
   As you are placing the precordial leads on her chest she states the fluttering has
   returned. Her vital signs are stable.

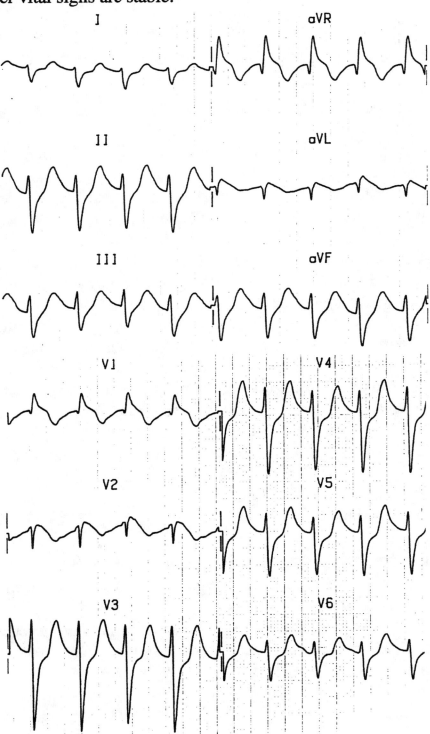

GLOSSARY OF TERMS

The words listed in this section are brief definitions of terms as they are used in this series and are not necessarily all-inclusive of the meaning of each word.

Aberrant - occasional abnormal intraventricular conduction of supraventricular impulses.

Accessory pathway - an abnormal conduction tract between the atria and ventricles.

Action potential - electrical changes in the myocardial cell membrane during the depolarization and repolarization of a cardiac cycle.

Activation - electrical stimulation of a portion of the heart.

Altered automaticity - an abnormal depolarization of cardiac cells.

Amplitude -the height of a waveform or complex measured in millimeters on the ECG graph paper.

Anterograde - electrical conduction of an impulse in a forward direction.

Antiarrhythmic - refers to medications that attempt to abolish, control or prevent dysrhythmias and ectopic impulses.

Arteriosclerosis - hardening of the arteries and loss of elasticity.

Atherosclerosis - a condition caused by an accumulation of debris along the intimal layer of arteries.

Atrial kick - normal contraction of the atria with movement of blood into the ventricles during diastole. This may account for as much as 25 percent of the total cardiac output.

Augment - to enhance or increase the size of the ECG tracing for better visibility.

Automaticity - the ability of a cell to depolarize spontaneously.

Automatic rate - the rate at which a dominant or escape pacemaker normally initiates electrical impulses.

Autonomic - the portion of the nervous system that involves the sympathetic and parasympathetic divisions that regulate involuntary body functions.

Axis - the position of the heart within the thoracic cavity.

Bigeminy - ectopic complexes occurring every other complex.

Bipolar - includes leads I, II and III. These leads record the potential between two points on the body. Also called the standard limb leads.

Bradycardia - a slow heart rate, typically less than 60 beats per minute.

Cannon waves - reflux waves of blood observed in the jugular veins when the atria contract against closed AV valves.

Capture - the appropriate timing of a pacemaker to depolarize the myocardium.

Cardiac output - the amount of blood pumped by the heart in one minute. Cardiac output is measured in liters per minute and can be calculated by multiplying the stroke volume by heart rate.

Chronotropic - influencing the heart rate.

Collateral circulation - microvascular connections that develop on the epicardium to improve blood supply to compensate for an insufficient supply of blood. These vessels develop in the presence of coronary artery disease.

Compensatory pause - a pause following a premature complex which allows the SA node to continue at its preset rhythm and regular R to R interval.

Complex - pertaining to the QRS waveforms and ventricular depolarization.

Conductivity - the property of cardiac cells to transmit electrical impulses.

Contractility - the ability of the cardiac cells to shorten when stimulated.

Controlled - a rhythm is considered to be controlled if the ventricular response is less than 100 beats per minute.

Couplet - two consecutive PVCs.

Cycle - one complete heartbeat including systole and diastole. A normal cycle includes the PQRST waveforms.

Demand - a pacemaker mode that initiates an impulse only upon failure of the atria or ventricles to fire within a preset time.

Depolarization - the electrical process of discharging a resting cardiac cell.

Diastole - period of relaxation of the atria and ventricles. It is during this phase that the chambers of the heart and coronary arteries fill with blood.

Differential - the correct diagnosis of a rhythm based on the exclusion or recognition of specific criteria.

Diphasic - refers to a single waveform that has two observable phases.

Dissociation - ocurrs when the pacemakers of the atria and ventricles are functioning independently. Sometimes called third degree AV block.

Dominance - term used to describe whether the left or right coronary artery supplies the greatest amount of blood flow to the base of the left ventricle.

Ectopic - a beat or rhythm originating from a site other than the SA node. Ectopic beats are often premature.

Equiphasic - pertaining to a QRS complex that is relatively equal in positive and negative deflections relative to the isoelectric line.

Escape - a complex or rhythm that is initiated when the underlying rhythm slows to less than the escape pacemaker's automatic rate.

Exclusion - diagnosis of a rhythm based on the fact that criteria for any other rhythm are not met.

Fascicle - pertaining to the intraventricular bundle branches.

Focus - the location from which an impulse arises.

Ground - electrode with a zero electrical potential that helps eliminate extraneous electrical interference.

Hemodynamic - the forces involved in perfusing the body with blood. Includes factors such as heart rate, force, preload and vessel tone.

Hexaxial - a reference system used to calculate the electrical axis of the heart. Each pole of any lead is divided into 30 degree sections.

Hypertrophy - enlargement of a portion of the heart without an increase in the chamber size. Hypertrophy is usually attributed to genetics or disease.

Infarction - necrotic tissue due to a sustained period of interrupted blood flow.

Infranodal - located within the SA or AV nodes.

Inherent - see automatic rate.

Injury - a portion of damaged myocardium capable of partial recovery.

Inotropic - influencing cardiac contractility and force.

Interpolated - a PVC landing precisely between two R waves. These beats do not have a typical compensatory pause.

Intraventricular - located within the ventricles.

Ischemia - reduced oxygenated blood flow to a portion of cardiac tissue which may be transient or reversible with early treatment and intervention.

Isoelectric - a flat line on the ECG graph indicating no electrical variations.

Joule - a unit of electrical energy delivered through the chest wall for the purpose of synchronized cardioversion or defibrillation of the heart.

MCL - modified chest lead. The bipolar chest leads of MCL1 and MCL6 simulate the precordial leads of V-1 and V-6.

Milliamps - a measurement of energy that is adjusted during cardiac pacing to elicit depolarization of the myocardium.

Mobitz - physician who identified the two types of second degree AV block.

Multifocal - term used to describe PVCs that originate from multiple locations.

Myocardium - pertaining to the heart muscle.

Necrosis - dead tissue from insufficient oxygenated blood flow.

Nodal - pertaining to the SA or AV nodes.

"No man's land" - extreme right or left axis deviation ranging from -91 to -179.

"Northwest quadrant" - see "no man's land."

Parasympathetic - the portion of the autonomic nervous system involved in slowing and depressing cardiac function.

Paroxysmal - sudden or abrupt onset of a dysrhythmia.

Pathologic - indicating a disease or abnormality.

Perpendicular - lead found at a 90 degree angle from a given lead. Identifying a perpendicular lead can be used to calculate the axis of the heart.

Plane - an anatomical view or angle of the heart.

Polarity - indicating a vector traveling toward a positive or negative lead.

Precipitating - factors or events that contribute to a condition or disease state.

Preload - a measurement of the amount of tension on the ventricular muscle fibers prior to contraction. Preload is directly related to end-diastolic blood volume.

Prime - a second abnormal waveform found within the same QRS complex.

Quadrigeminy - ectopic beat occurring every fourth complex.

"Rabbit ears" - refers to an RSR' QRS configuration.

Reciprocal - refers to ECG changes observed in an opposite lead.

Reentry - a source of ectopic beats caused by a single electrical impulse reentering a portion of tissue for a second or subsequent time.

Refractory - inability to respond to an electrical stimulus.

Repolarization - the process by which a cell is restored to a ready state.

Retrograde - the flow of electrical current opposite the normal direction.

Stroke volume - the amount of blood pumped by the left ventricle each beat.

Supraventricular - refers to any portion of the heart from the bundle branches to the SA node.

Sympathetic - the portion of the autonomic nervous system involved in stimulating cardiac activity.

Symptomatic - adverse signs or symptoms related to a dysrhythmia or disease.

Synchronize - an electrical shock timed to depolarize the myocardium during the R wave. This prevents depolarization during the vulnerable T wave.

Systole - contraction and subsequent movement of blood through the ventricles.

Tachycardia - a rapid heart rate, typically greater than 100 beats per minute.

Threshold - a measurement of sensitivity of response to a stimulus.

Thrombolytic - a substance that breaks down or dissolves a thrombus.

Thrombosis - a blood clot within a vessel that has the potential to restrict flow.

"Tombstone T wave" - a hyperacute T wave resembling the shape of a tombstone. These T waves are often seen early in the development of an MI and are usually associated with ST elevation.

Trancutaneous - refers to pacing patches applied to the skin of the chest wall.

Transmural - pertaining to an infarcted area penetrating through the full thickness of the myocardium.

Transvenous - an internal pacemaker inserted directly into the heart via a vein.

Trigeminal - an ectopic complex arising every third beat.

Triggered activity - condition in which the myocardial cells depolarize more than once following a single impulse.

Triphasic - a single waveform that has three observable phases.

Uncontrolled - a term used to describe a rhythm with a ventricular response greater than 100 per minute.

Unifocal - arising from a single ectopic focus.

Unipolar - electrical activity measured from the positive electrode to the zero reference point located in the center of the heart.

Vagal - refers to the tenth cranial (vagus) nerve that influences heart rate and AV node conduction by regulating parasympathetic tone.

Vector - the magnitude and direction of a wave of depolarization.

Viable - pertaining to the ability to live or be resuscitated.

Voltage - the height or depth of a waveform measured in millimeters.

Wenckebach - physician credited with discovering second degree AV block type I.

COMMON CARDIAC MEDICATIONS

Antiarrhythmic Agents

Class I - Fast Sodium Channel Blockers

A.   Quinidine
     Procainamide
     Disopyramide

B.   Lidocaine
     Mixiletine
     Phenytoin
     Tocainide

C.   Flecainide
     Propafenone

Class II - Beta Blockers

Atenolol
Esmolol
Metoprolol
Propranolol
Timolol

Class III - Prolongs Refractory Period

Bretylium
Amiodarone

Class IV - Calcium Channel Blockers

Diltiazem
Nifedipine
Verapamil

Potassium Channel Opener

Adenosine

Analgesics
Narcotics
- Morphine
- Meperidine
- Fentanyl
Sedatives
- Diazepam

Anticoagulants
Aspirin
Heparin
Coumarin derivatives

Diuretics
Carbonic anhydrase inhibitors
- Acetazolamide
Loop Inhibitors
- Ethacrynic acid
- Furosemide
Potassium sparing agents
-Spironolactone
Osmotics
- Mannitol
Thiazides
- Hydrochlorothiazide

Electrolyte Replacement
Calcium
Magnesium
Potassium
Sodium

Negative Inotropic Agents
Beta Blockers
Calcium Channel Blockers

Parasympathetic Blocking Agent
Atropine

Positive Inotropic Agents

Digitalis Glycosides
- Digoxin

Sympathomimetic Agents
- Amrinone
- Dobutamine
- Dopamine
- Epinephrine
- Isoproterenol
- Norepinephrine

Thrombolytic Agents

Altepase (tPA)
Anistreplase (APSAC)
Streptokinase
Urokinase

Vasodilators

Beta Blockers
Calcium Channel Blockers
Nitrates
- Isosorbide
- Nitroglycerin
Nitroprusside

CARDIAC ASSESSMENT

A thorough cardiac assessment requires a strong knowledge of cardiovascular anatomy and physiology. It also involves learning a variety of hands-on skills. Listed below is a brief outline to help you organize your class sessions.

History

History of Current Illness

O - when was the *onset* of symptoms?
P - what *provoked* the symptoms?
Q - what is the *quality* of the symptoms?
R - does the pain *radiate* anywhere?
- does anything provide *relief*?
- do the symptoms occur at *rest*?
S - how *severe* are the symptoms?
T - *timeframe* - are the symptoms constant or intermittent?

History of Past Illnesses and Surgeries

Medications
current medications
allergies
compliance

Hereditary Factors

Environmental Factors

Lifestyle
substance or tobacco use
stress
exercise/rest
nutrition
weight

Physical Exam

General Appearance and Affect
anxiety
restlessness

Vital Signs
blood pressure, pulse and respirations

Skin Signs
color
turgor
temperature
capillary refill
moisture
edema
clubbing

Veins
jugular volume
cannon waves
varicosities
hepatojugular reflux

Arteries
central and peripheral pulses
mean arterial pressure

Chest Wall
excursion
symmetry

Heart Sounds
murmurs
gallops
splits

<u>Lung Sounds</u>
    crackles
    wheezes
    friction rubs

<u>Oxygenation Status</u>
    cough/sputum
    respiratory effort
    work of breathing

Diagnostic Studies

<u>Routine Studies</u>
    serum
        - lipids
        - enzymes
        - coagulation
        - electrolytes
        - medication levels
    urine
    12-lead ECG
    pulse oximetry
    arterial blood gases
    chest X-ray

<u>Special Studies</u>
    cardiac catheterization and angiography
    radionuclide testing
    electrophysiology studies
    hemodynamic monitoring
    positron emission tomography
    magnetic resonance imaging

Other Systems

In addition to a complete cardiac assessment, it is important to assess for potential disorders in other systems. Cardiac problems can be exacerbated by diseases involving other body systems. Also, keep in mind that medications prescribed for non-cardiac diseases may have a direct effect on the cardiovascular system.

Liver

Endocrine
>   diabetes
>   thyroid
>   adrenal
>   pituitary

Renal
>   urine output
>   failure

Gastrointestinal
>   bleeding

Cerebrovascular
>   syncope
>   history of stroke

Neurological
>   level of consciousness

Sensory/Perception

Psychological
>   compliance with prudent lifestyle
>   coping ability

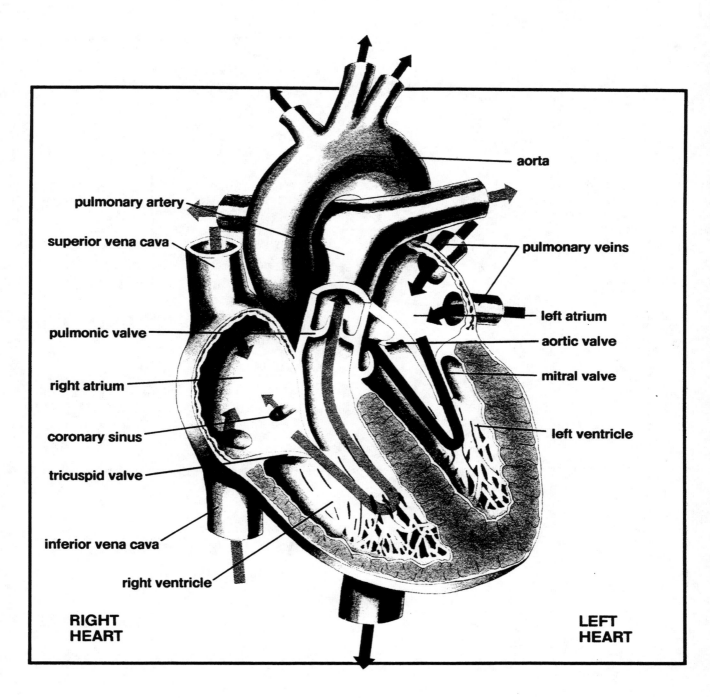

Fig. 1-1.

Circulation of blood through the heart

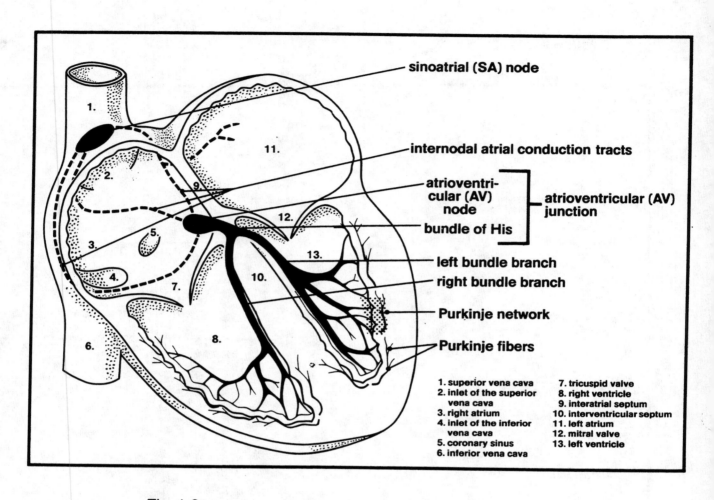

Fig. 1-2.

Electrical conduction system of the heart

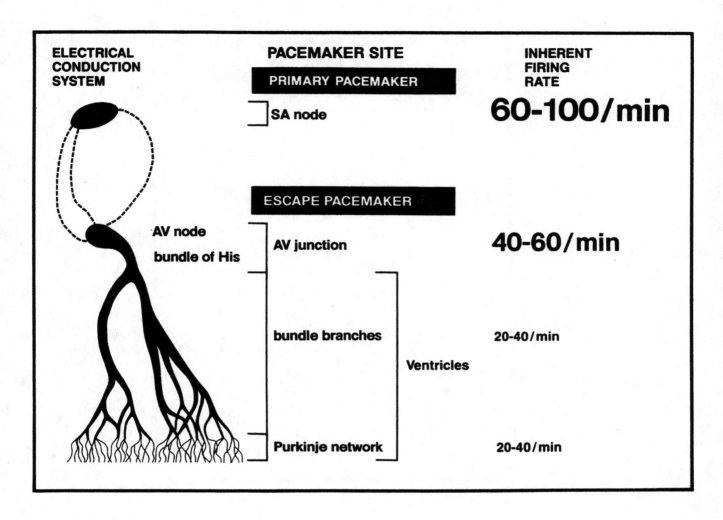

Fig. 1-3.

Primary and escape pacemakers of the heart

Rate Conversion Table

Small Squares	Heart Rate Per Minute	Small Squares	Heart Rate Per Minute
4	375	21	72
5	300	22	68
6	250	23	65
7	214	24	63
8	188	25	60
9	168	26	58
10	150	28	54
11	136	30	50
12	125	32	47
13	115	34	44
14	107	36	42
15	100	38	40
16	94	40	38
17	88	42	36
18	83	44	35
19	79	48	31
20	75	50	30

Fig. 1-4

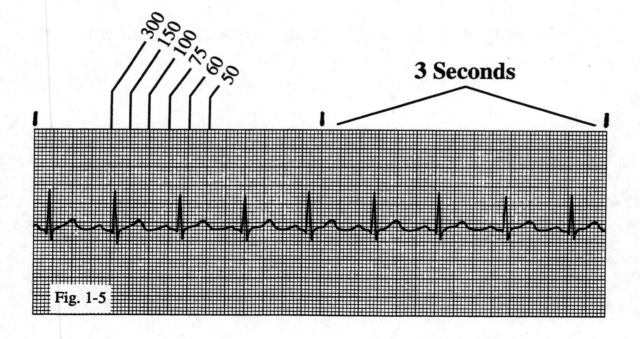

Fig. 1-5

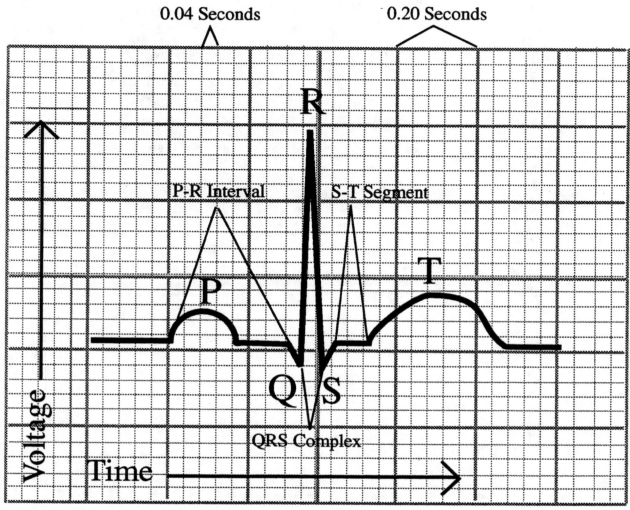

Fig. 1-6

Components of the ECG Tracing

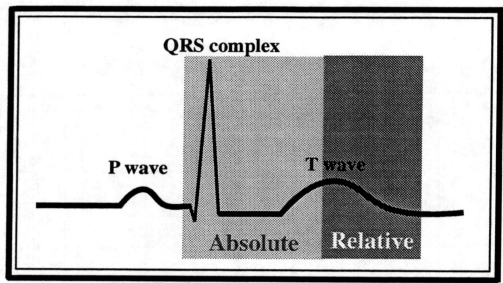

Fig. 1-7   **Refractory Periods**

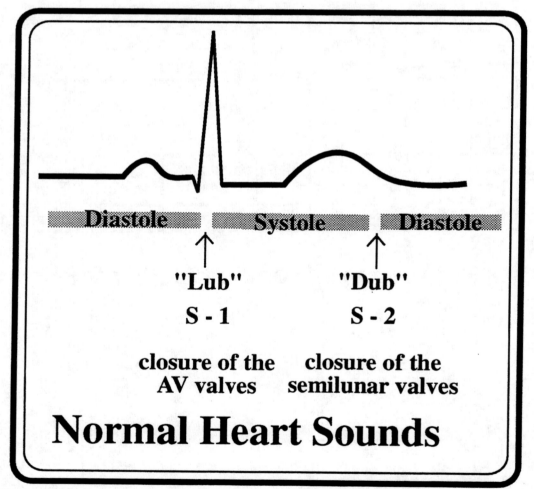

Normal Heart Sounds

Fig. 1-8

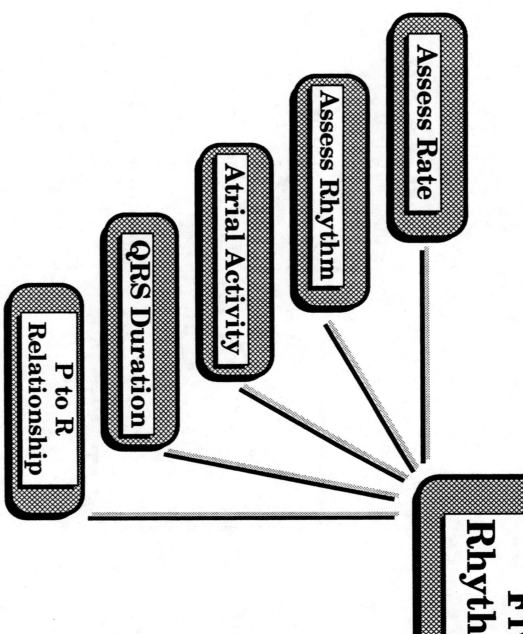

Assess Rate

Assess Rhythm

Atrial Activity

QRS Duration

P to R
Relationship

Five Step
Rhythm Analysis

Fig. 1-9

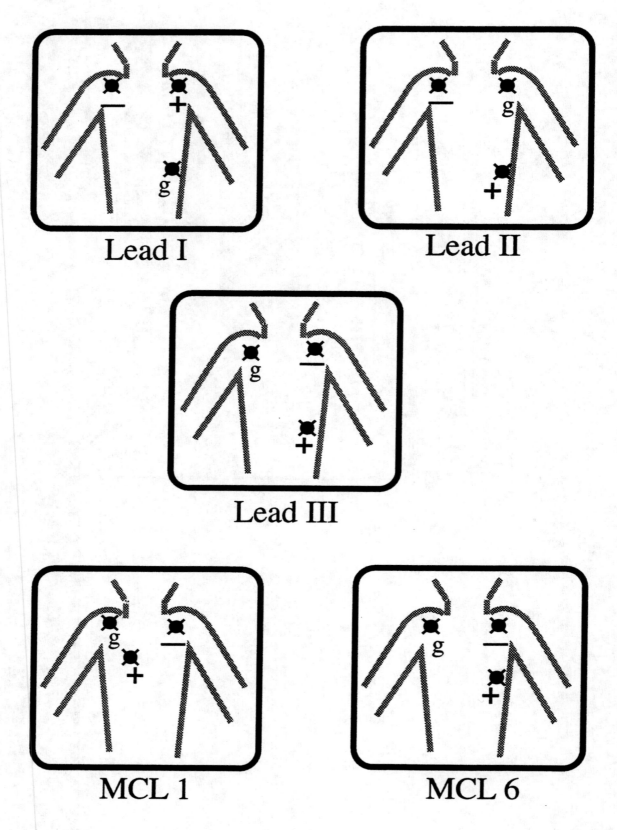

Lead I

Lead II

Lead III

MCL 1

MCL 6

Fig 1-10

ECG Troubleshooting

Artifacts are distortions that obscure the cardiac impulse on the ECG tracing. Artifact may be caused by electrical, mechanical or patient interference. This often makes accurate interpretation difficult. Artifact may appear similar to a life threatening dysrhythmia. Remember, the "patient is always right". Be sure to check the status of your patient before initiating any electrical or drug therapy. Listed below are a few tips for eliminating unwanted artifact:

Patient Preparation

Explain procedure
Preserve modesty
Dry skin
Remove hair
Gently abrade and clean skin
Insure personal and patient safety

Check for and correct

Amplitude of gain
Lead selection
Dry electrode gel
Loose electrodes
Lead wire connection
Damage to lead wires
Improper electrode placement
Patient movement
T wave amplitude greater than R wave
60-cycle interference

Fig. 1-11

AV JUNCTION

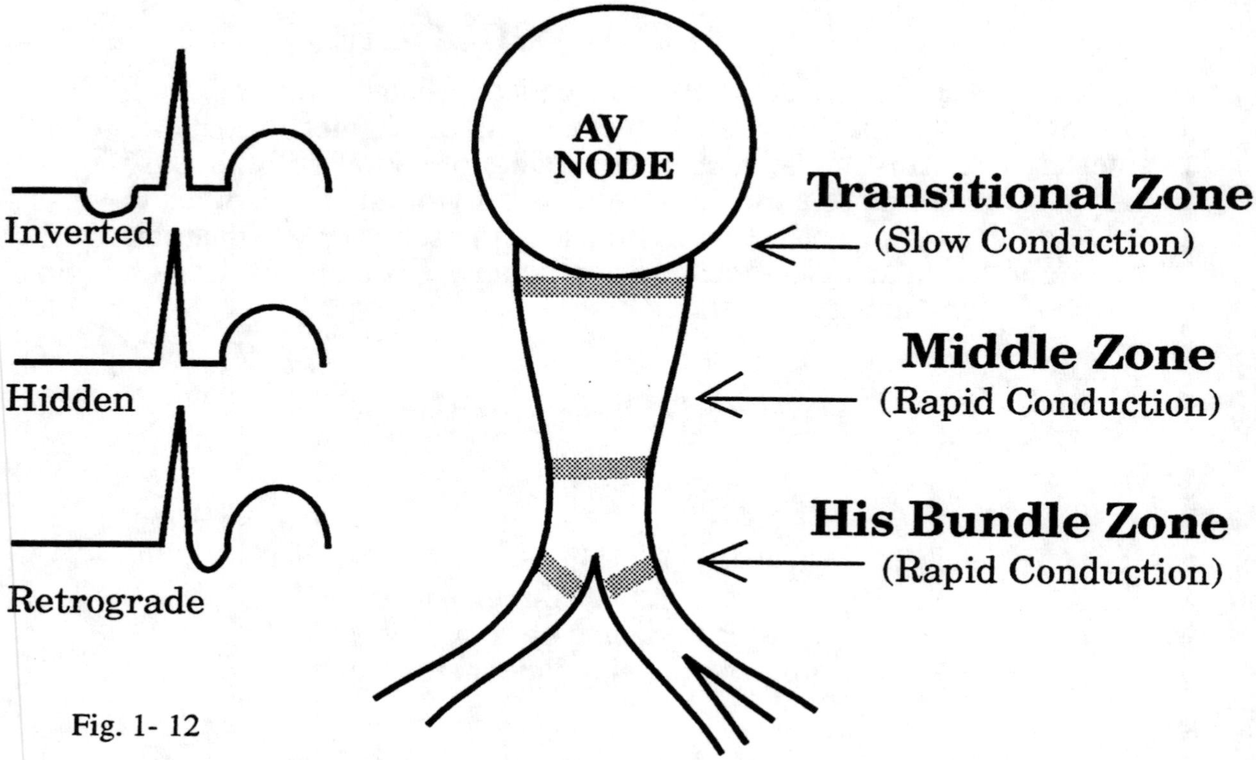

Inverted

Hidden

Retrograde

Fig. 1- 12

AV
NODE

Transitional Zone
(Slow Conduction)

Middle Zone
(Rapid Conduction)

His Bundle Zone
(Rapid Conduction)

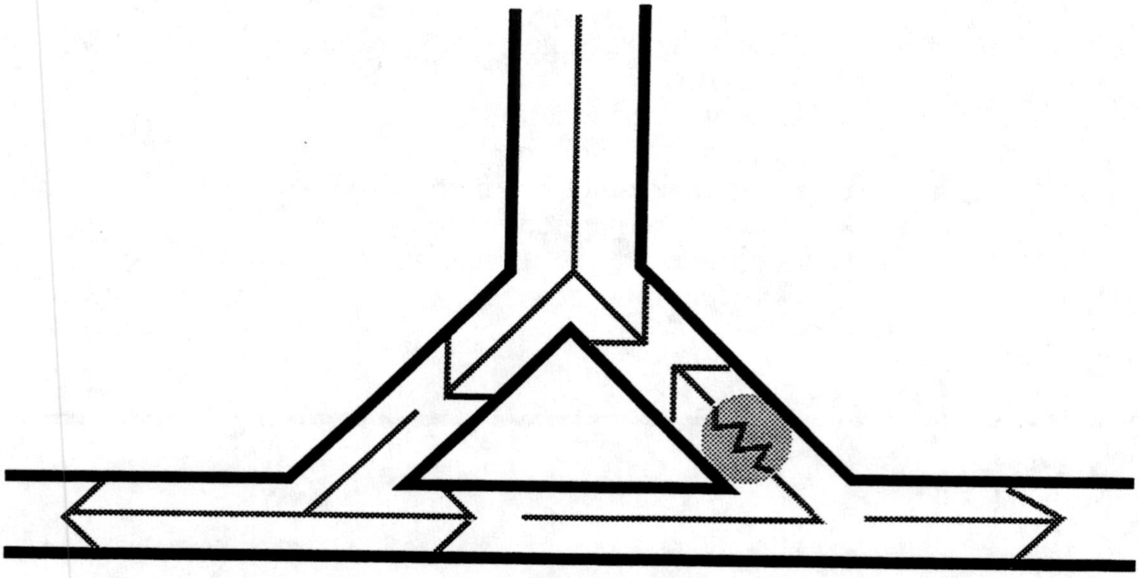

Fig. 1-13

REENTRY

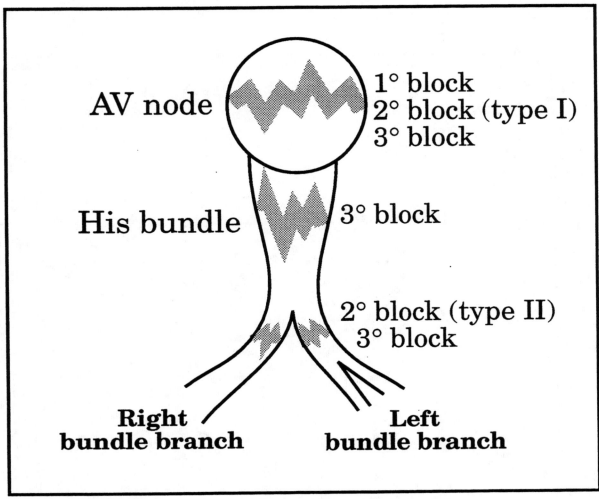

Fig. 1-14   **Locations of AV blocks**

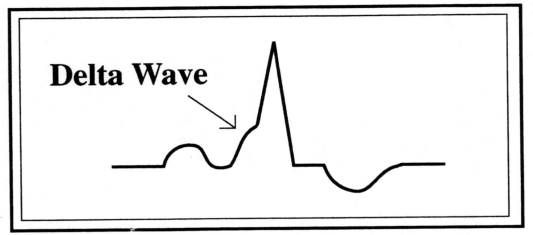

Fig. 1-15

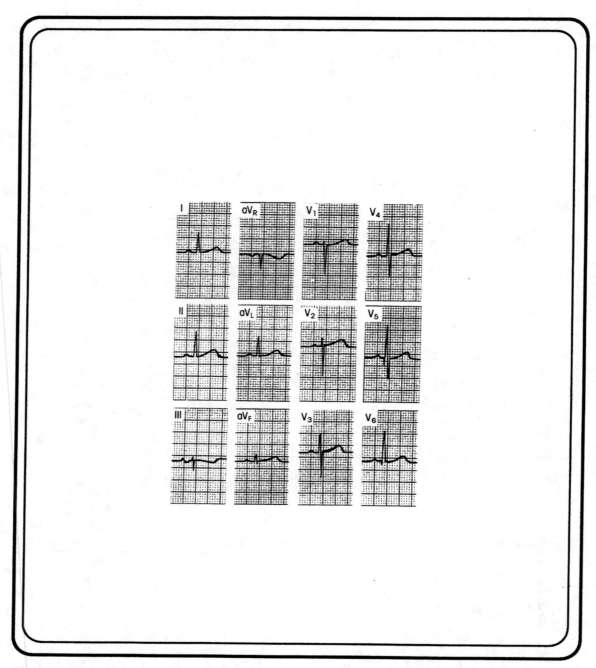

Fig. 1-16   **The Normal 12-lead ECG**

Standard Limb Leads (Bipolar)

I	Lateral Wall
II	Inferior Wall
III	Inferior Wall

Augmented Limb Leads (Unipolar)

aVR	Non-Specific View
aVL	Lateral Wall
aVF	Inferior Wall

Precordial Chest Leads (Unipolar)

V1	Anteroseptal Wall
V2	Anteroseptal Wall
V3	Anterior Wall
V4	Anterior Wall
V5	Lateral Wall
V6	Lateral Wall

Fig. 1-17

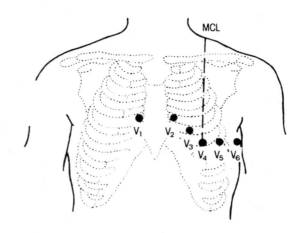

Precordial Chest Leads

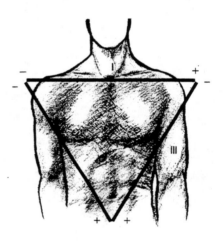

Einthoven's Triangle

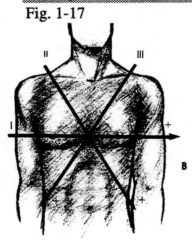

Bipolar Limb Leads

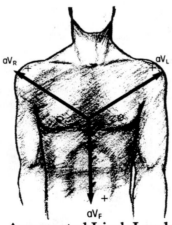

Augmented Limb Leads

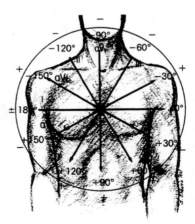

Hexaxial Reference System

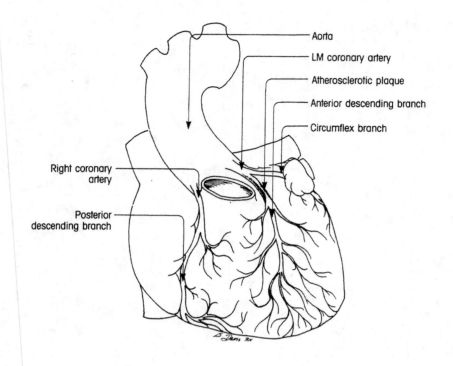

Aorta

LM coronary artery

Atherosclerotic plaque

Anterior descending branch

Circumflex branch

Right coronary artery

Posterior descending branch

Fig. 1-18

The Coronary Arteries

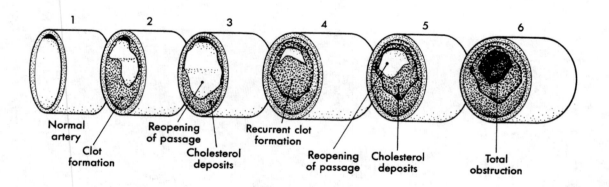

1

2

3

4

5

6

Normal artery

Clot formation

Reopening of passage

Cholesterol deposits

Recurrent clot formation

Reopening of passage

Cholesterol deposits

Total obstruction

Fig. 1-19

Coronary heart disease and atherosclerosis

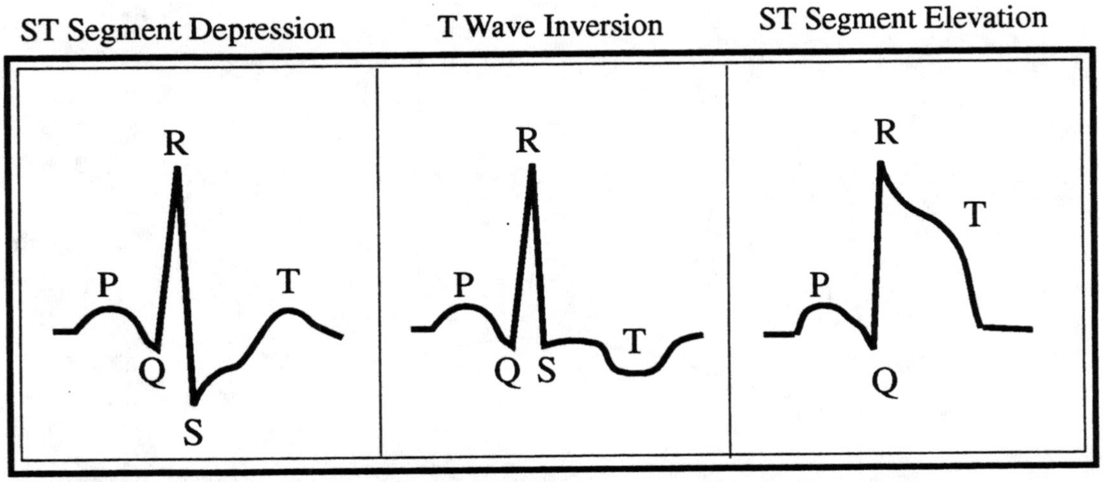

ST Segment Depression   T Wave Inversion   ST Segment Elevation

Fig. 1-20 **ECG Changes Associated With Ischemia**

The three major causes of a myocardial infarction are:

- the formation of a blood clot in a coronary artery
- a hemorrhage beneath a layer of plaque
- a dislodged segment of plaque

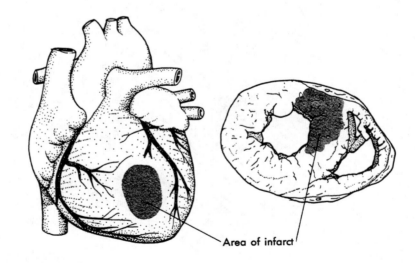

Area of infarct

Fig. 1-21

Acute myocardial infarction

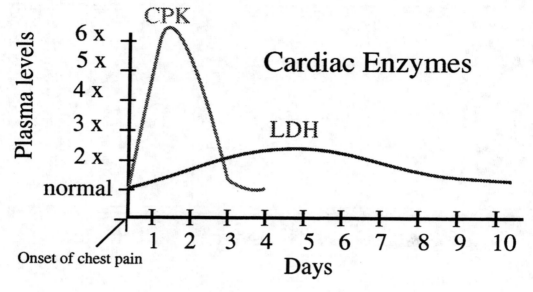

Fig. 1-22

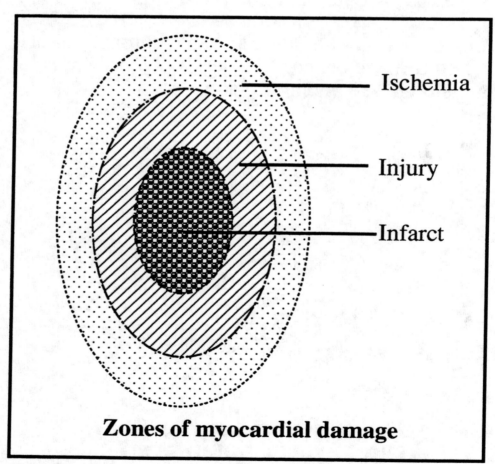

Fig. 1-23

ANNOTATED BIBLIOGRAPHY

MOSBY TEXTS

Acute Coronary Care, 2nd Edition.
Califf, Mark and Wagner, 1993. A comprehensive guide to current treatment of myocardial infarction. Emphasis is placed on providing state-of-the-art care through all phases of treatment. Recommended for instructor or advanced student level.

Atrial Arrhythmias: Curent Concepts and Management
Touboul and Waldo, 1991. An advanced, highly technical text focused on the the recognition and management of atrial rhythms. Topics include pathophysiologic mechanisms, electrophysiologic studies and catheter ablation.

Basic Dysrhythmias: Interpretation and Management.
Huszar, 1988. A simply written, well illustrated text designed to assist the beginning student acquire the skills required to recognize common dysrhythmias. The clinical significance and treatment of each dysrhythmia is discussed. Includes 223 practices rhythms.

Cardiovascular Nursing: Holistic Practice
Dossey and Guzzetta, 1992. This text focuses on assessment, diagnosis and treatment of adult patients with medical and surgical cardiovascular dysfunctions. Emphasis is placed on the holistic approach to treatment and care.

Cardiovascular Physiology, 6th Edition.
Berne and Levy, 1992. This book is designed for the student seeking an in-depth presentation of cardiovascular physiology. Topics include electro-physiology, regulation of heartbeat, coronary circulation and hemodynamics.

Comprehensive Cardiac Care, 7th Edition.
Kinney, Packa, Andreoli and Zipes, 1991. A detailed review of the latest information related to diagnosis and treatment of cardiovascular disorders. A useful text for learners at all levels.

Early Defibrillation

Huszar, 1991. A basic text intended to be used as a guide for training in the use of automated external defibrillators. Useful for individuals working in the prehospital or emergency setting.

Myocardial Infarction, 4th Edition.

Goldberger, 1991. A comprehensive text that provides a detailed review on the 12-lead elctrocardiographic diagnosis of myocardial infarction. Recommended for the instructor or advanced student level.

Thrombolysis: Basic Contributions and Clinical Progress.

Haber and Brunwald, 1991. A collection of writings from over 40 authors covering the current body of knowledge and future trends in thrombolysis.

Understanding Electocardiography: Arrhythmias and the 12-Lead ECG, 6th Edtion.

Conover, 1992. A sequential presentation of the principles and criteria necessary to accurately interpret 12-lead ECGs. An excellent resource for the beginning to advanced student.

MOSBY SLIDES

Fundamentals of the 12-lead ECG

Cooper and Marriott, 1987. 50 Slides and guide.

Arrhythmias and Blocks

Cooper, 1987. 50 slides, guide and workbook.

Ventricular and Supraventricular Arrhythmias

Marriott, 1984. 112 slides and guide.

Arrhythmias - Know the Causes

Marriott, 1988. Slides, guide and workbook.

Ventricular Ectopy Vs. Aberration

Marriott, 1988. 64 slide and guide.

Intermediate-Advanced 12-Lead ECG.

Marriott, 1987. 114 slide and guide.

VIDEOS

American Safety Video Publishers, Inc.

Automated Defibrillation
(VHS 30 minutes)

ACLS Skills Review
(VHS 30-45 minutes each)
8 tape series includes:
> Airway management
> IV Procedures
> ECG Recognition
> Arrhythmia Interpretation
> Conversion Techniques
> Pharmacology One
> Pharmacology Two
> Mega Code
> Instructor's Manual

Mosby-Yearbook

The Wide QRS Complex Tachycardia: Differential Diagnosis
Marriott, 1986.
(VHS 55 minutes)